American Public Health Association
VITAL AND HEALTH STATISTICS MONOGRAPHS

Accidents and Homicide

Accidents and Homicide

ALBERT P. ISKRANT / PAUL V. JOLIET

1968 / HARVARD UNIVERSITY PRESS

Cambridge, Massachusetts

PREFACE

In this work we are taking advantage of the more accurate population data around 1960 than in noncensus years, and the mortality rates calculated for the three-year period 1959, 1960, and 1961, to estimate the extent of accident and homicide problems with accuracy and to describe some relations of the statistics available as well as trends in accidental death rates. We present here also, as precisely and completely as possible, the current stage of knowledge regarding factors associated with specific types of accidents, hypotheses regarding causes of accidents, and methods that could be used in controlling accidental injuries and deaths.

The sources of data include special tabulations prepared by the National Center for Health Statistics on mortality from accidents and homicide, presented as rates in the Appendix. The second group of tables was obtained from statistics on injuries for the period July 1959-June 1961, also prepared by the National Center for Health Statistics. We have presented some of these figures in the Appendix following the mortality rates but have not included statistics available in publications of the National Health Survey: these are from the old National Health Survey Series B and the new Series 10 of the National Center for Health Statistics.

For the period July 1959-June 1961 special questions were included in the National Health Survey on "type of accident"; the data therefrom are presented in their publications Series B (Nos. 37, 39, 40, 41, and 42) and in the Appendix of this book. Throughout the text all published figures from the National Health Survey Series B are referenced as "National Health Survey." Tables 1 through 59 in the Appendix are referred to as "Appendix Table 1, etc." Mortality data not included in the Appendix are referenced as publications of the National Center for Health Statistics. All data refer to the United States unless otherwise noted.

In this manuscript the term Division of Accident Prevention will refer to that Division of the Public Health Service, now no longer existent. A reorganization has assigned the functions of the Division to the Injury Control Program of the National Center for Urban and Industrial Health.

We have received much assistance from personnel of the Division of Accident Prevention in assembling, editing, and reviewing this material, and we should like to thank all members of the Division for their cooperation. In particular, the staff of the Epidemiology and Surveillance Branch has helped substantially in various ways to make this monograph a reality.

Albert P. Iskrant
Paul V. Joliet, M.D., M.P.H.

CONTENTS

TABLES

CHARTS

FOREWORD

Rapid advances in medical and allied sciences, changing patterns in medical care and public health programs, an increasingly health-conscious public, and the rising concern of voluntary agencies and government at all levels in meeting the health needs of the people necessitate constant evaluation of the country's health status. Such an evaluation, which is required not only for an appraisal of the current situation, but also to refine present goals and to gauge our progress toward them, depends largely upon a study of vital and health statistics records.

Opportunity to study mortality in depth emerges when a national census furnishes the requisite population data for the computation of death rates in demographic and geographic detail. Prior to the 1960 census of population there had been no comprehensive analysis of this kind. It seemed appropriate, therefore, to develop for intensive study a substantial body of death statistics for a three-year period centered around that census year.

A detailed examination of the country's health status must go beyond an examination of mortality statistics. Many conditions such as arthritis, rheumatism, and mental diseases are much more important as causes of morbidity than of mortality. Also, an examination of health status should not be based solely upon current findings, but should take into account trends and whatever pertinent evidence has been assembled through local surveys and from clinical experience.

The proposal for such an evaluation, to consist of a series of monographs, was made to the Statistics Section of the American Public Health Association in October 1958, and a Committee on Vital and Health Statistics Monographs was authorized. The members of this Committee and of the Editorial Advisory Subcommittee created later are:

Committee on Vital and Health Statistics Monographs

Mortimer Spiegelman, Chairman
Paul M. Densen, D. Sc.
Robert D. Grove, Ph.D.
Clyde V. Kiser, Ph.D.
Felix Moore
George Rosen, M.D., Ph.D.

William H. Stewart, M.D. (withdrew June 1964)
Conrad Taeuber, Ph.D.
Paul Webbink
Donald Young, Ph.D.

Editorial Advisory Subcommittee

Mortimer Spiegelman, Chairman
Duncan Clark, M.D.
E. Gurney Clark, M.D.
Jack Elinson, Ph.D.

Eliot Freidson, Ph.D. (withdrew
February 1964)
Brian MacMahon, M.D., Ph.D.
Colin White, Ph.D.

The early history of this undertaking is described in a paper that was presented at the 1962 Annual Conference of the Milbank Memorial Fund.[*] The Committee on Vital and Health Statistics Monographs selected the topics to be included in the series and also suggested candidates for authorship. The frame of reference was extended by the Committee to include other topics in vital and health statistics than mortality and morbidity, namely fertility, marriage, and divorce. Conferences were held with authors to establish general guidelines for the preparation of the manuscripts.

Support for this undertaking in its preliminary stages was received from the Rockefeller Foundation, the Milbank Memorial Fund, and the Health Information Foundation. Major support for the required tabulations, for writing and editorial work, and for the related research of the monograph authors was provided by the United States Public Health Service (Research Grant CH 00075, formerly GM 08262). Acknowledgment should also be made to the Metropolitan Life Insurance Company for the facilities and time that were made available to Mr. Spiegelman, now retired from its service, who proposed and administered the undertaking and served as general editor. The National Center for Health Statistics, under the supervision of Dr. Grove and Miss Alice M. Hetzel, undertook the sizable tasks of planning and carrying out the extensive mortality tabulations for the period 1959-1961. Dr. Taeuber arranged for the cooperation of the Bureau of the Census at all stages of the project in many ways, principally by furnishing the required population data used in computing death rates and by undertaking a large number of varied special tabulations. As the sponsor of the project, the American Public Health Association furnished assistance through Dr. Thomas R. Hood, its Deputy Executive Director.

[*]Mortimer Spiegelman, "The Organization of the Vital and Health Statistics Monograph Program," *Emerging Techniques in Population Research* (*Proceedings of the 1962 Annual Conference of the Milbank Memorial Fund;* New York: Milbank Memorial Fund, 1963), p. 230. See also Mortimer Spiegelman, "The Demographic Viewpoint in the Vital and Health Statistics Monographs Project of the American Public Health Association," *Demography,* Vol. 3, No. 2 (1966), p. 574.

Because of the great variety of topics selected for monograph treatment, authors were given an essentially free hand to develop their manuscripts as they desired. Accordingly, the authors of the individual monographs bear full responsibility for their manuscripts, and their opinions and statements do not necessarily represent the viewpoints of the American Public Health Association or of the agencies with which they are affiliated.

Berwyn F. Mattison, M.D.
Executive Director
American Public Health Association

NOTES ON TABLES

1. Regarding 1959-1961 mortality data:
   a. Deaths relate to those occurring in the United States (including Alaska and Hawaii);
   b. Deaths are classified by place of residence (if pertinent);
   c. Fetal deaths are excluded;
   d. Deaths of unknown age, marital status, nativity, or other characteristics have not been distributed into the known categories, but are included in their totals;
   e. Deaths were classified by cause according to the *Seventh Revision of the International Statistical Classification of Diseases, Injuries, and Causes of Death* (Geneva: World Health Organization, 1957);
   f. All death rates are average annual rates per 100,000 population in the category specified, as recorded in the United States census of April 1, 1960;
   g. Age-adjusted rates were computed by the direct method using the age distribution of the total United States population in the census of April 1, 1940 as a standard.[1]
2. Symbols used in tables of data:
   - - - Data not available;
   . . . Category not applicable;
   - Quantity zero;
   0.0 Quantity more than zero but less than 0.05;
   * Figure does not meet the standard of reliability of precision:
       a) Rate or ratio based on less than 20 deaths;
       b) Percentage or median based on less than 100 deaths;
       c) Age-adjusted rate computed from age-specific rates where more than half of the rates were based on frequencies of less than 20 deaths.
3. Geographic classification:[2]
   a. Standard Metropolitan Statistical Areas (SMSA's): except in the New England States, "an SMSA is a county or a group of contiguous counties which contains at least one city of 50,000 inhabitants or more or 'twin cities' with a combined population of at least 50,000 in the 1960 census. In addition, contiguous counties are included in an SMSA if, according to specified criteria, they are (a) essentially metropolitan in character and (b) socially and economically integrated with the central city or cities."

---

[1] Mortimer Spiegelman and H. H. Marks, "Empirical Testing of Standards for the Age Adjustment of Death Rates by the Direct Method," *Human Biology,* 38:280 (September 1966).
[2] *Vital Statistics of the United States,* 1960 (Washington, D.C.: National Center for Health Statistics, 1963), Vol. 2 (*Mortality*), Part A, Section 7, p. 8.

In New England, the Division of Vital Statistics of the National Center for Health Statistics uses, instead of the definition just cited, Metropolitan State Economic Areas (MSEA's) established by the Bureau of the Census, which are made up of county units.

b. Metropolitan and nonmetropolitan: "Counties which are included in SMSA's or, in New England, MSEA's are called metropolitan counties; all other counties are classified as nonmetropolitan."

c. Metropolitan counties may be separated into those containing at least one central city of 50,000 inhabitants or more or twin cities as specified previously, and into metropolitan counties without a central city.

4. Sources:

In addition to any sources specified in the figures, text tables, and appendix tables, the deaths and death rates for the period 1959-61 are derived from special tabulations made at the National Center for Health Statistics, Public Health Service, U. S. Department of Health, Education, and Welfare, for the American Public Health Association.

Accidents and Homicide

1 / INTRODUCTION

Man has a persistent tendency to tamper with his environment and so lives in one of his own making, frequently without anticipating the consequences. Abel Wolman has pointed out that deaths and injuries from accidents "are perhaps excellent examples of the real challenges to public health of the future, because inherent in them, are the intertwined practices and mores of the entire way of life of the present century."[1] John Gordon also has emphasized the complexity of public health today due to man's alteration of his environment, and has stated that "the departures from health, are mainly manmade. They result from the things man does to himself and what he does to his environment."[2] A much greater threat than any intrinsic in the struggle of man against nature lies in the expansion of that intellectual activity itself which has led man to create new dangers much more formidable and deadly than those caused by nature or by the animal species, forgotten by evolution. The pressure now comes from our own biologic success as a species. Newspapers may highlight deaths due to tornadoes in the Middle West or to hurricanes in the South and East; but the grim fact is that on any weekend more persons are killed on the highways by motor vehicles than are killed by the forces of nature.

The increasing significance of accidents

Throughout school, early workyears, and early days of marriage, a person in the United States is more likely to die from an accident than from any other cause; and throughout life as a whole, accidents are outranked as a cause of death only by the cardiovascular diseases and by cancer. Accidental injuries have become the leading cause of death in young people—not because accidents have been on the increase, but because other causes of death have decreased. The increase in relative significance of accidents in young people is illustrated in Chart 1.1, which shows what proportion of all deaths have been due to accidents since the beginning of the century. From 1900 to date the increase in this proportion in the age group 15-24 is of particular importance. Accidents now cause almost 60 percent of the deaths in that age group; among men, motor vehicles alone cause over 40 percent.

The trend in death rates from what in 1900 were the five leading

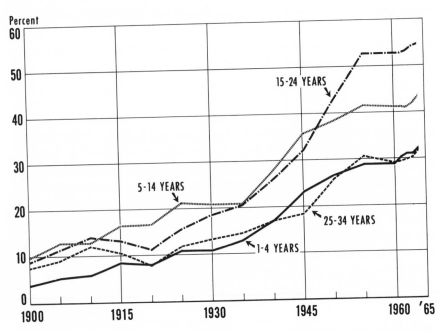

Chart 1.1 Deaths from all accidents as a percentage of all deaths for persons aged 1-34 years: United States, 1900-1964. Source: Division of Vital Statistics, National Center for Health Statistics.

causes of death in the four age groups under 35 is depicted in Charts 1.2, 1.3, 1.4, and 1.5. These show that accidental injuries have remained a leading cause of death; but the other four causes important in 1900 have practically disappeared or have declined considerably. It will be noted that in the age group 25-34, heart disease alone remains a challenge to accidental injuries as a leading cause of death. In the age group 15-24, accidental deaths have shown not only a relative increase in rate, but also an absolute increase—to a large extent the result of the dramatic increase in deaths from automobiles.

The public health problem of accidental injuries cannot be confined to the subject of death. Accidents also cause impairment, disability, hospitalization, loss of days from work or school, and so on. Throughout this monograph it will be emphasized that what is included in the term "accidents" will depend on the use to be made of the information or data being collected. If the subject is accidental deaths in the United States, the discussion is confined to statistics on deaths; if the subject is causes of hospitalization, use is made of data regarding accidental injuries that result in hospitalization. If the subject is injuries that need treatment by a physician, the information comes from physicians, hospitals, out-patient departments, clinics and others involved with the treatment of injuries.

Sources and purposes of accident data

Mortality data are produced by the Division of Vital Statistics of the National Center for Health Statistics of the Public Health Service from tabulations of data from all death certificates in the United States. Additional information is sometimes obtained by the Division of Accident Prevention of the Public Health Service, through the use of supplements to the death certificate and through actual investigation of the circumstances surrounding incidents of death. Data on

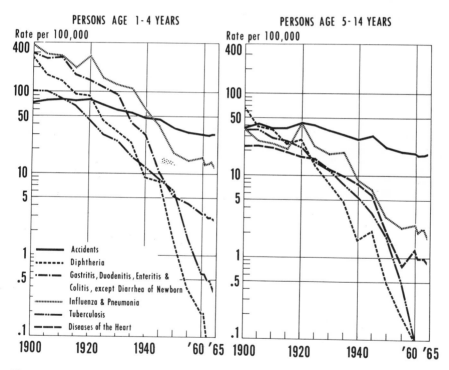

Charts 1.2 (*left*) and 1.3 (*right*). Death rates for the five leading causes of death in 1900 for persons aged 1-4 years and for persons aged 5-14 years: United States, 1900-1964. Source: Division of Vital Statistics, National Center for Health Statistics.

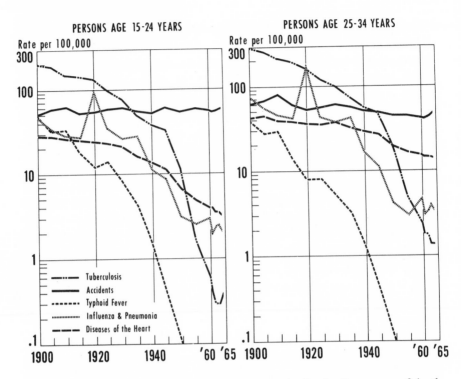

Charts 1.4 (*left*) and 1.5 (*right*). Death rates for the five leading causes of death in 1900 for persons aged 15-24 years and for persons aged 25-34 years: United States, 1900-1964. Source: Division of Vital Statistics, National Center for Health Statistics.

accidental injuries in the United States are developed in gross through the National Health Survey of the National Center for Health Statistics, and estimates are made of the incidence of accidental injuries in the nation and in broad geographic areas. Current gross estimates of deaths and injuries from accidents are made and published annually by the National Safety Council in a booklet entitled *Accident Facts* using preliminary data submitted from various sources. More refined information for special localities is obtained through reporting systems instituted by the Division of Accident Prevention, health departments in some areas, and other sources. Sometimes the reporting of accidental injuries is limited to hospitalized cases, sometimes it includes out-patient departments, and occasionally it involves the cooperation of private physicians. Again, the purpose for which the data are intended determines the kind of information to be collected and the period it should cover.

In general, data on accidental injuries and deaths are obtained for one of the following purposes: estimation of the extent and nature of a problem in a particular area; provision of information for program planning regarding types and circumstances of the causes of accidental injuries; collection of information to establish baselines where programs or projects of prevention are to be evaluated; and provision of individual cases on which additional information can be obtained. The detail obtained on one particular incident, again, depends on the purpose for which the information is to be used; but in general the place of the accident, the type of accident, the nature of the injury, and a certain amount of information regarding the circumstances under which the accident occurred are included.

The possibility of bias (because of the different characteristics of patients) through reporting by particular types of treatment sources should be borne in mind; when income groups are compared, data from the National Health Survey sometimes show differences among the groups in the frequency of medically treated injuries and injuries causing disability.

Sometimes accidental injury information is obtained through sample household surveys—the National Health Survey uses this method—and sometimes local groups conduct surveys. An example of the latter is a survey dealing with farm and farm home accidents carried out in cooperation with the University of Missouri.[3] A survey has also been made in Connecticut as part of a research grant from the Public Health Service.[4] Problems of recall—depending on the severity of the injury—and the ability of persons being questioned to respond for other members of the household create difficulties in such interviews that are discussed in publications of the National Health Survey.

One of the problems involved in the reporting of accidental injuries is the classification system to be used. In general, deaths are tabulated by the E-code of the International Classification of Diseases, which categorizes type of accident according to the agent involved (motor vehicle, fire) and the action (fall, submersion) resulting in injury or death. Data on injuries collected by the National Health Survey have a somewhat different classification. This is partly because the types of accidents that cause death most frequently are not always the types that cause most injuries. In Chapter 4, where the data are presented by type of accident, this difference of classification will be obvious.

Annual estimates of "disabling" injuries occurring in the United States are made and published by the National Safety Council. In general these estimates are based on activity restriction and are much lower than the estimates of all injuries made by the National Health Survey. These differences are discussed in *Accident Facts.*[5]

Another problem that arises in the comparison of statistics is the denominator to be used in the calculation of rates. It has been traditional in the industrial safety movement to calculate injury rates on the basis of man-hours of exposure. This practice has been followed by the National Safety Council and other organizations in calculating rates of death and injury from motor vehicle and other transport accidents where the estimated number of miles traveled has been considered the base. It is often necessary to introduce the concept of population "at risk," especially where comparison is made of the effect of variables on rates. Throughout the present work rates are those based on resident population, not population "at risk" or other measures of exposure, unless otherwise specified.

The scope of the accident problem in general

In Chapter 4, data for the years 1959-1961 are used to express both the problem of deaths and that of injuries, because this is the period for which the population bases for rates are most reliable (derived as they are from the census of 1960), and for which detail on types of accidental injuries is available. Changes have occurred since then, especially in motor-vehicle deaths; the three-year average of most recent data, therefore, is presented as the best estimate of the extent of the current injury problem. Estimates of the annual toll of accidental injuries for the period 1963-1965 are:

Persons killed	104,000
Working years of life lost	2,000,000
Persons injured	52,000,000
Bed-disabled	11,000,000
Having received medical care	45,000,000
Hospitalized	2,000,000
Days of restricted activity	512,000,000
Days of bed-disability	132,000,000
Days of work loss	90,000,000
Days of school loss	11,000,000
Hospital bed-days	22,000,000

The last five items in the foregoing tabulation are for days lost on account of impairments and current injuries.

It is estimated that 65,000 hospital beds and 88,000 hospital personnel are needed at present for the treatment of injuries, and that the prevalence of impairments caused by injuries is over 11,000,000.

Of accidental deaths, about 40 percent are caused by motor vehicles, 20 percent by falls, 8 percent by fire and explosion, 7 percent by drowning, and 2-3 percent by firearms (see Appendix Table 10).

Of injuries, about 27 percent are caused by falls, 9 percent by having been struck by a moving object, 8 percent by having bumped into an object or person, and 6 percent by moving motor vehicles or cutting or piercing instruments (National Health Survey).

Each year in the United States over 500,000,000 days of restricted activity are the result of accidental injuries, or about 17 percent of restricted activity from all medical causes. Accidental injuries are the leading cause of days of restricted activity because of acute (short-term) conditions; the second greatest cause is the common cold. Over 130,000,000 of these days are considered bed-disabling; these are about 12 percent of all days spent in bed because of medical conditions. About 90,000,000 days of work loss (over 20 percent of all work loss) and over 11,000,000 days of school loss are caused by injuries.

About 2,000,000 persons are hospitalized for injuries each year, which is almost 10 percent of all admissions to general hospitals and 12 percent of all admissions excluding deliveries. These injury admissions result in about 22,000,000 hospital bed-days; they are the leading cause of bed-days in general hospitals, exceeding even deliveries, and they exceed the total of three other leading causes—heart conditions, cancer, and diabetes.

In addition to deaths and the disability involved in current injuries, a more permanent kind of health problem is created by impairments due to injuries. It is estimated that there are about 11,000,000 impairments due to injuries in the noninstitutional population in the United States—a rate of 60 per 1,000 persons. These cases constitute 16 percent of all visual impairments, 15 percent of paralysis, 76 percent of absences of major extremities, and 57 percent of impairments of limbs, back, and trunk. Approximately 2,000,000 of these 11,000,000 impairments are considered serious enough to prevent each person involved from pursuing the major activities of his age-sex group.

The 11,000,000 impairments include 500,000 visual impairments. Injuries are the single leading cause of visual impairment in persons under 65 years of age; this impairment, further, is more common in males than females. About 400,000 impairments of hearing are due to injury, with the highest proportion caused by injuries in the age group 25-44; again, the rate of such impairments is higher in males than in females.

About 200,000 persons have lost major extremities because of accidental injuries; the rate in this category is much higher in males than in females. In males about 84 percent of amputations are caused by injuries.

Over 7,500,000 people have impairments involving limbs, back, or trunk, and in every age group more of these impairments were caused by injury than by all other causes combined. The rate of such impairments is higher in males than in females.

Of the impairments due to injury, over one-fourth result from accidents described as falls, and in persons 65 years of age or over almost 40 percent are from falls; moving motor vehicles are responsible for about 15 percent. Of the impairments due to injury sustained at work, over one-fourth are the result of accidents involving machinery in operation; this is in fact almost 12 percent of all impairments due to injury. A type of accident that does not have much influence on the death rate but is important as a cause of impairment is described as "one-time lifting or exertion" and accounts for approximately 600,000 impairments in the United States.[6]

Because accidents are the greatest cause of death in the younger years of life, the accumulated work-loss years attributable to accidents exceeds the total attributable to any other cause. (The years from age 15 to 65 are considered working years.) Altogether, somewhat over 13,000,000 working years of life are lost each year by premature death; 2,000,000 such years are lost through death from accidental injuries—approximately 15 percent of the total. Accidents are followed in order by heart disease and cancer as a cause of working years lost.

The death rate from accidents has declined gradually from a peak in 1936, the year that the highest number of accidental deaths was recorded to date (110,052: a rate of 85.4 per 100,000 persons). The corresponding figures for 1960 were, approximately, 94,000 deaths: a rate of 52 per 100,000. The peak in 1936 was in part caused by the gradual increase in deaths from motor vehicles without a compensating decline in the number of deaths from all other accidents—this even though there had been a gradual decline over the years in the death rate from non-motor-vehicle accidents. A secondary peak occurred in 1941, again due to a drastic increase in motor-vehicle accidental deaths—which reached a rate of 30 per 100,000. This rate has not been reached since. From 1941 to 1942 there was a precipitous decrease in the death rate from motor-vehicle accidents, coincident with the participation of the United States in World War II. At the end of the war there was again an increase in the death rate for motor-vehicle accidents, but it never quite returned to the prewar level. The death rate from non-motor-vehicle accidents showed a rather steady and continuous decline from 1943 to 1960. In older persons the decline has been noteworthy; this is discussed in Chapter 3, in the section entitled "Accidents to the Aged". The downward trend is also discussed in parts of Chapters 3 and 4.

Beginning in 1962 there was a rather substantial increase in the number of deaths and corresponding rates from causes involving motor vehicles—an increase which has continued into 1966. No corresponding increase in the death rate for non-motor-vehicle accidents is evident (see Chart 1.6).

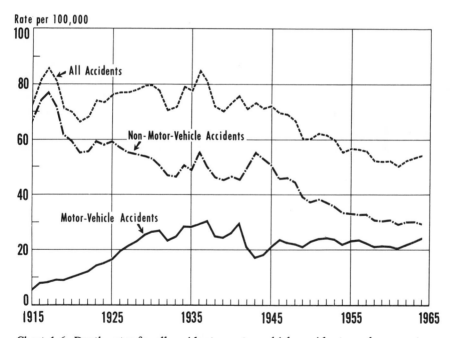

Chart 1.6. Death rates for all accidents, motor-vehicle accidents, and non-motor-vehicle accidents: United States, 1915-1964. Source: Division of Vital Statistics, National Center for Health Statistics.

Accidents in the Armed Forces

Observation of the large body of personnel in the Armed Forces, made up mostly of men and women in the prime of life working under special situations, yields an accident picture different from that of the civilian population. Comparisons of the accident experiences of the civilian and military populations are affected not only by obvious differences in age and sex composition, but also by differences in marital status, living arrangements, and activities.

In 1960, there were 2,971 accidental fatalities and 89,563 admissions to hospitals for nonbattle injury among military personnel on active duty in the three services combined. The number of deaths from accidental causes was approximately three-quarters of the total number of deaths in each of the three services.[7]

Mortality and morbidity statistics concerning the Armed Forces are published independently by the Office of the Surgeon General of each branch of the services.[8] Because of the consequent differences in extent and comparability of the data, appropriate references must be consulted before using data for comparative purposes.

For all Naval personnel, the accident death rate decreased from 150 per 100,000 strength in 1950 to 140 per 100,000 strength in 1960. The rate in the Air Force also declined, from 226 per 100,000 strength in 1951 to 118 in 1960. The trend of the accident death rate in the Army is not very clear because of changes in definition and coverage. The rates for the Army were 173 and 110 per 100,000 strength in 1950 and 1960, respectively.

About 50 percent of all deaths due to injuries in the Armed Forces are the result of motor-vehicle accidents—for the most part accidents on civilian highways. The motor-vehicle death rate in all three services decreased from the 1950's to 1960. The rate for the Army declined from 78 per 100,000 strength in 1950 to 59 in 1960. After 1960, however, the rate for the Army increased to 71 per 100,000 strength (1964). The rate in the Navy also declined from the 1950's to 1960: it was 80 per 100,000 strength in 1950 and 60 in 1960. The motor-vehicle death rate has shown a pronounced trend in the Air Force: 73 per 100,000 strength in 1951, it was 56 in 1960 and 44 in 1965. The Air Force recently conducted a countermeasure experiment as part of a program toward prevention of motor-vehicle accidents. During the year in which the countermeasure was applied there was a significant reduction in accidents.[9]

The nonbattle-injury hospital-admission rates decreased for all three services from 1950 to 1960. These rates for the Army, Navy, and Air Force were, respectively, 76, 44, and 45 per 1,000 strength in 1950 (1951 for the Air Force), and 49, 27, and 30 per 1,000 strength in 1960. (A change of definition occurred in the Army between 1950 and 1960.)

The motor vehicle is the leading cause of nonbattle-injury admissions in all three services—about 22 percent in the Air Force, 25 percent in the Navy, and about 15 percent in the Army in 1960. In all services, injuries from athletics and sports and from machinery and tools account for a rather high percentage of the injuries treated.

Accidental deaths in various countries

An insight into mortality from accidents and motor-vehicle accidents in various countries is provided by a report of the World Health Organization for the period 1960-1962 (Table 1.1).[10] Accident mortality in a particular country reflects in large measure the economy, culture, and mores of that country; it is, in addition, influenced to some extent by definitions. In motor-vehicle accidents the level of mortality is closely related to the use of motor vehicles.[11]

Among these countries with the highest rates for all accidents are Chile, Austria, France, the United Arab Republic, South Africa, and Switzerland. The United Arab Republic and Chile have high rates in spite of the fact that the death rate from motor-vehicle accidents is extremely low in these countries. On the other hand, the motor-vehicle death rate is high in South Africa, Austria, Germany, Australia, Switzerland, and the United States and Canada. For non-motor-vehicle transport accidents the death rates are highest in Norway; Finland and Hungary follow.

Low accident death rates are found in the Dominican Republic, Singapore, Hong Kong, El Salvador, Ceylon, and Israel, all of which have low rates for motor-vehicle fatalities.

Scotland has the highest death rate from poisoning of any country with pertinent records, followed by Austria, Finland, Poland, and England and Wales. The city of West Berlin has the highest death rate from falls, but it is an entirely urban area. Switzerland leads among nations in deaths from falls, followed by Austria, Denmark, Norway, Sweden, and Germany.

Deaths from fire and explosion are extremely high in the United Arab Republic and exceed by far the death rates of any other country. Others with high rates include the United States, Portugal, Colombia,

Table 1.1 Death rates for specified types of accidents and homicide: selected countries, 1960-62

Country	All accidents (AE138-AE147)	Motor-vehicle (AE138)	Other transport (AE139)	Poisoning (AE140)	Falls (AE141)	Machinery (AE142)	Fire and explosion (AE143)	Hot substance, etc. (AE144)	Firearm (AE145)	Drowning (AE146)	All other accidents (AE147)	Homicide (AE149)
South Africa	60.7	27.3	3.0	1.7	6.9	0.6	3.6	0.6	0.7	6.5	9.8	----
United Arab Republic	61.2	2.6	2.0	0.7	3.2	0.1	14.2	0.6	0.0	6.4	31.4	----
Canada	53.3	20.9	3.2	2.0	9.0	1.3	3.3	0.3	1.2	4.9	7.2	----
Chile	71.9	7.6	----	----	----	----	----	----	----	----	----	----
Colombia	48.9	8.6	1.1	1.5	7.2	0.1	3.8	0.1	0.4	8.9	17.2	----
Costa Rica	34.3	6.1	----	----	----	----	----	----	----	----	----	----
Dominican Republic	17.4	4.6	----	----	----	----	----	----	----	----	----	----
El Salvador	27.7	6.8	0.7	1.1	7.0	0.1	1.4	0.6	0.9	4.2	4.9	----
Guatemala	34.0	9.2	----	----	----	----	----	----	----	----	----	30.3
Mexico	39.9	3.1	----	----	----	----	----	----	----	----	----	----
Panama	34.4	5.4	1.2	1.6	4.2	0.5	1.7	1.3	1.4	6.6	10.5	----
Puerto Rico	32.2	9.2	0.5	0.5	5.4	0.5	1.6	0.2	0.5	5.0	8.8	----
Trinidad and Tobago	31.3	14.6	1.8	0.5	3.3	0.5	1.1	1.1	0.3	4.3	3.8	----
United States	51.7	21.2	2.3	1.7	10.5	1.1	4.0	0.2	1.3	2.9	6.5	4.7
Venezuela	43.0	16.3	1.2	1.1	4.6	0.3	2.6	1.2	1.8	5.9	8.0	7.3
Ceylon[a]	29.2	2.0	----	----	----	----	----	----	----	----	----	----
Hong Kong	23.6	5.4	2.1	0.7	3.9	0.1	1.2	1.0	0.0	5.5	3.7	----
Israel[b]	29.8	9.0	----	----	----	----	----	----	----	----	----	----
Japan[a]	43.5	11.6	4.6	1.4	4.4	0.5	1.6	0.4	0.1	7.6	11.3	----
Singapore	21.2	8.4	0.6	0.6	2.8	-	-	0.9	0.1	4.0	3.8	----

	1	2	3	4	5	6	7	8	9	10	11	12
Austria	66.7	26.5	4.0	4.3	18.6	0.7	0.9	0.8	0.2	3.5	7.2	1.2
Belgium	53.3	18.7	1.0	2.1	9.1	0.2	0.4	0.4	0.1	2.9	18.4	0.6
Czechoslovakia	47.9	13.6	3.9	2.9	11.5	0.5	1.1	0.3	0.4	3.8	9.9	--
Denmark	46.7	17.7	2.7	2.8	18.0	0.2	0.8	0.1	0.2	1.7	2.5	0.5
Finland	54.1	17.9	5.4	4.2	12.3	0.5	1.4	0.4	0.8	6.8	4.4	--
France	62.5	19.1	1.3	2.8	14.5	0.1	0.3	1.4	0.5	5.4	17.1	--
Germany[c]	57.6	26.0	2.5	1.4	16.9	0.9	0.5	0.8	0.2	2.1	6.2	--
West Berlin	50.5	13.1	1.2	2.7	28.7	0.2	0.6	0.8	-	1.2	2.0	1.2
Greece	31.2	5.1	1.1	1.3	9.2	1.1	0.4	1.6	1.0	3.3	7.1	--
Hungary	34.9	6.7	5.3	1.6	10.1	0.3	1.2	0.3	0.7	2.8	5.9	--
Ireland	32.4	8.8	1.7	1.0	9.2	0.2	0.9	1.6	0.3	5.0	3.7	--
Italy[a]	41.2	17.3	2.2	1.1	11.5	0.2	0.8	0.8	0.4	2.9	4.0	--
Netherlands	39.2	17.9	2.6	1.0	10.5	0.4	0.5	0.3	0.1	3.3	2.6	0.3
Norway	47.1	9.0	7.5	1.7	17.9	0.3	0.5	0.2	0.6	5.3	4.1	--
Poland	33.9	4.5	4.4	3.2	1.2	0.2	0.5	0.6	0.2	3.9	15.2	--
Portugal	39.5	9.6	3.2	1.0	8.6	0.3	3.9	0.9	0.5	7.7	3.8	0.9
Spain	30.1	6.7	1.7	0.9	4.4	0.6	0.4	0.8	0.5	3.0	11.1	--
Sweden	45.7	14.3	3.7	1.6	17.0	0.4	1.1	0.1	0.5	2.9	4.1	0.6
Switzerland[a]	60.4	21.2	3.9	2.5	19.3	0.5	0.8	0.8	0.5	3.9	7.0	--
England and Wales	38.6	14.3	1.4	3.2	11.9	0.5	1.4	0.2	0.2	1.9	3.6	0.5
Northern Ireland	35.3	12.1	0.7	2.1	9.8	0.7	2.8	0.6	0.4	2.3	3.8	0.8
Scotland	47.9	13.4	2.3	5.4	13.5	0.4	2.3	0.2	0.2	3.7	6.4	0.7
Australia	52.2	25.5	2.9	1.7	8.7	0.8	2.0	0.3	1.0	3.9	5.4	1.5
New Zealand[a]	43.1	13.1	3.6	1.7	12.8	1.6	1.1	0.3	0.8	3.4	4.7	--

Note: Death rates for each type of accident were obtained by applying the percentage distribution by type in a single year to the rate for that year for "all accidents." AE numbers are from an alternate that is less detailed than the standard E-code.

Source: Demographic Yearbook, 1962 (United Nations: New York, 1962), tables 4 and 5; Epidemiological and Vital Statistics Report (World Health Organization: Geneva, 1965), 18:117–124; and unpublished tabulation of accident mortality by type of accident and homicide according to age, sex, and selected country.

a. 1959-61
b. Jewish population only
c. Federal Republic

and South Africa. It may be mentioned parenthetically that the death rate from fire and explosion among nonwhites in the United States approaches that of the United Arab Republic and is higher than for any other country.

Firearm deaths are highest in Venezuela, Panama, the United States, and Canada. Deaths from drowning are highest in Colombia, Portugal, and Japan, but Finland, Panama, South Africa, and the United Arab Republic also have high rates.

In general, accident death rates are higher for males than for females. A few notable exceptions appear: in Hong Kong the deaths from non-motor-vehicle transportation are the same for males and females; in Scotland the death rate for poisoning is as high for females as for males. Death rates for falls are higher for males than females except in European countries and countries of European stock. This phenomenon (probably due to fractured hips) will be discussed more fully in the sections entitled "Accidents to the Aged" (Chapter 3) and "Falls" (Chapter 4).

Some countries have extremely high rates for the category "all other" accidents. These rates are, presumably, due to accidents from causes not as universal as those usually specified. The United Arab Republic, Belgium, Colombia, France, and Poland are among such countries.

Different methods of classifying causes of death may account for differences in death rates between various countries. But Scotland and Canada are noteworthy for high accident death rates in infants; this phenomenon does not occur among older children, whose rates are lower. It also is interesting to note differences in the rates of those killed *in* the automobile and those killed *by* the automobile while pedestrians. Italy, Scotland, Ireland, and Japan have high proportions of motor-vehicle pedestrian deaths.

There is no consistent pattern in the change of death rates from accidents between the period around 1950 and the period around 1960. Some countries have shown increases and others have shown decreases. For motor-vehicle fatalities, however, the picture is different: nearly all countries—with the notable exception of the United States—have shown increases, some of which have been rather large.

2 / EPIDEMIOLOGY

In this monograph, the definition of MacMahon and others of epidemiology as "the study of the distribution and determinants" of accidental injuries in man will be used.[1] The focus will be on identification of factors associated with accidental injuries for the purpose of formulating hypotheses and identifying causes in the hope, ultimately, of developing public health programs that can reduce the frequency of accidental injuries or ameliorate their effects.

In considering the epidemiology of accidents, Gordon talks about interaction of the host, agent, and environment.[2] Data will be presented under those three headings in the following chapters. The person injured or killed in the accident will be considered the "host"; the type of accident will be a generalization of the "agent"; and such elements as the place of the accident and other physical and social environmental factors will be included in the "environment." There is, of course, some common ground among the three factors; for purposes of simplification, social factors will be included in the category "host" rather than "environment."

The definition of an accident, and what is included in the epidemiology of accidents, is important. It is our opinion that in searching for clues to causation it is essential to clarify the degree of injury for which clues are sought. In carrying out studies of the characteristics of people who are "accident prone" this point is often not considered. The assumption of a continuum from mild injury to death to which the same principles of prevention apply may often be unwarranted: when the causes of fatal accidents or accidents that create injuries necessitating hospitalization are investigated, the characteristics of both people and circumstances may differ from those observed when one investigates minor injuries requiring only a brief visit to a physician or the application of local medication. (Haddon, Suchman, and Klein, however, seem to express the contrary point of view in their discussion of "accident-behavior."[3]) The severity of an injury or the likelihood of death varies with the type of accident, the circumstances under which it occurred, and the characteristics of the person injured. With this in mind, it is reasonable to include both deaths and injuries in any investigation of particular accidents.

We recognize that many factors are involved in the causation of accidents, whereas certain diseases—especially communicable ones—are caused by a single germ or agent. It is the opinion in some quarters that the search for accident causes is a hopeless pursuit because accidents may be the indirect outcome of a group of circumstances rather than the direct result of a single determinant. The epidemiologic approach to the causation of accidents offers real hope for the derivation of meaningful hypotheses that will lead to realistic programs of prevention. One great advantage of investigations of accidental injuries and deaths is that usually there is no incubation period; the injury or death occurs either simultaneously with the accident or within a very short period thereafter.

Because of this multiplicity of factors, the team approach to the investigation of incidents is gaining increased acceptance. The Division of Accident Prevention of the Public Health Service is establishing such teams in different demographic areas of the United States. The team approach involves the acquisition of specific information by persons with different skills; perhaps its greatest advantage is the interaction allowed between members of each team as they discuss their findings and attempt to develop hypotheses of causation.

In describing the problem of accidental deaths and injuries or the factors affecting them, one is immediately faced with the diverse approaches to this problem—both in program planning and in research. There is some interest, for example, in carrying out research or developing programs of prevention for the preschool child, for children in general, or for the aged. This approach is based on the fact that characteristics of the host (like the supervision given a child, or the failing senses of an elderly person) comprise a particular segment of the program that can be studied as a separate entity, regardless of the type of accident or the agent involved. (A discussion of such factors is included in Chapter 3.)

On the other hand, there is interest in accidental deaths and injuries from the point of view of the type of accident involved. Deaths are classified by the Public Health Service and other organizations under the E-code of the International Classification of Diseases described in Chapter 1. There are in existence some research or prevention programs concerned with deaths and injuries caused by falls or by fire and explosion. This approach to the problem is presented in Chapter 4.

Still another approach concerns the place in which an accident might occur: there are, for example, conferences on home accidents, research projects into their causes, and groups organized to develop programs for their prevention. There is also interest in accidental injuries that occur under such broad headings as recreation or industry.

This approach, to place of accident, is probably the most common of the four. The structure of the National Safety Council has been very influential in promoting this classification of accidents, discussed in Chapter 5.

Other approaches to the problem begin with the traumatic injury or the nature of the injury (Chapter 6). Obviously, for example, fractures can occur in motor-vehicle accidents, in fires, from falls, or in almost any type of traumatic accident.

In general, the present discussion will focus on data on mortality from the special tabulations prepared for 1959-1961, and at times on other mortality data, data from the National Health Survey on the incidence of accidental injuries, and data from special studies and surveys conducted by the Division of Accident Prevention of the Public Health Service and by other organizations. From these special investigations, impressions regarding factors associated with accidents and tentative hypotheses that can be tested in studies specially designed for the purpose will be presented.

There will be some repetition, necessary for readers interested in any one of the four approaches mentioned above, of items discussed in the following chapters. As an extreme example, the matter of a possible relation in elderly people between bone conditions and fractures from falls will be touched on in the sections "Accidents to the Aged," "Falls," "Home," and "Physical and Medical Conditions" (in Chapters 3, 4, and 5). Nevertheless, an attempt has been made to keep duplication to a minimum.

3 / HOST FACTORS

Certain characteristics of people, and the hazards to which they expose themselves by the ways in which they live, are in large part responsible for accidental deaths and injuries. There are obvious differences in the types of accidents that occur to men and to women, and to persons of different ages. For instance, injuries resulting from accidental ingestion of poisonous substances are largely the problem of young children; and the death rate from automobile accidents is highest among persons in their late teens and early twenties and much higher in males than in females. Factors in the host do not in themselves determine types or frequency of accidents, but they do contribute to probability of occurrence.

Factors with less obvious effects on frequency and types of accidental injuries include marital status, race (color), geographic location, income, education, family size, housing, and occupation. Still less clear are the effects of such social factors as customs, influence of peer groups, social status, role changes (changes in marital status or employment, for example), major life disruptions, and other social and sociopsychological factors. It would be impossible to discuss all the hypotheses and theories that have been developed regarding the effects of particular host factors on accidental injuries. In the sections that follow, reference is made to several of the factors most commonly discussed; some available statistics are also presented.

Age

From at least two points of view, age is an important factor in the problem of accidental death and injury. As might be expected, the various types of accidents occur with different frequencies in different age groups; furthermore, the case fatality rate varies with age and is generally highest in the very young and the old. The curve of the death rate from a particular type of accident, by age, is a function of the incidence of injuries due to that type of accident and the chance of survival once injury occurs.

The age distribution for deaths differs with accident type, but for accidents in general it is a somewhat J-shaped curve: high in infants under one year, low in teenagers and young adults, increasing steadily with age (see Chart 3.1). The injury rate for males is in the opposite pattern: low for the preschool child and the elderly and extremely high for teenagers and young males (Chart 3.2). This results in a ratio of injury to death that is low at both extremes of life and high in

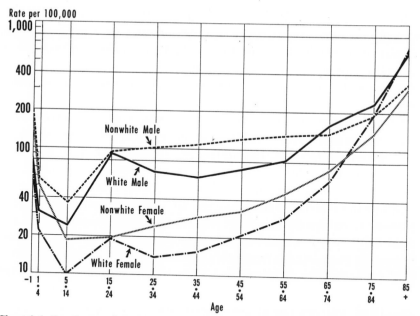

Chart 3.1. Death rates for all accidents by age, color, and sex: United States, 1959-1961.

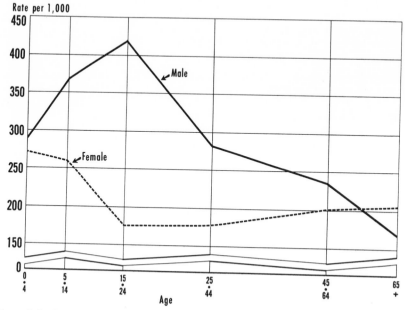

Chart 3.2. Rates for all injuries by age and sex: United States, July 1959-June 1961. Source: Division of Health Interview Statistics, National Center for Health Statistics.

school children (Chart 3.3). Stated differently, the case fatality rate is high at both extremes of life and lowest in school children. Ratios of injury to death are higher for females than for males at all ages. The drop in ratios in the age group 15-24, especially for males, is due to a high case fatality rate for motor vehicles and firearms in that group.

The general similarity of the age distributions of deaths from falls, fires, and motor-vehicle accidents to pedestrians illustrates problems that are associated with immaturity and fragility at both extremes of life. Conversely, death rates from motor vehicles (nonpedestrian deaths), drowning, firearms, and other activities associated with recreation show peaks in males in their late teens and early adult years. Injuries from machinery occur most frequently to adult males, and that death rate is highest among persons in their fifties and sixties; moreover, these injuries frequently involve amputation. As mentioned earlier, death from accidental poisoning by ingestion is essentially the problem of the preschool child, whereas that from gases and vapors is associated with persons in their later years.

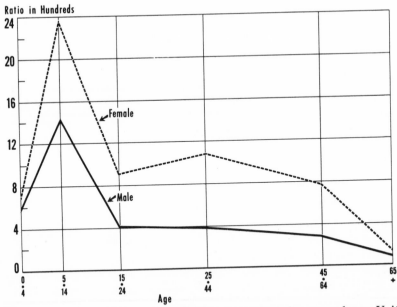

Chart 3.3. Ratio of injuries to deaths for all accidents by age and sex: United States, 1959-1961. Sources: deaths—Division of Vital Statistics, National Center for Health Statistics, 1959-1961; injuries—Division of Health Interview Statistics, National Center for Health Statistics, July 1959-June 1961.

Many of these differences in patterns are discussed in the sections on specific accident types. Because of the peculiar problems of accidental injuries in children and in the aged, there are separate discussions for these groups. Other considerations of age are included in the sections on sex and color.

Childhood accidents. There are nearly 56,000,000 children under 15 years of age in the United States; each year more than 15,000 of them die from accidents, a rate of about 28 per 100,000. Another 17,000,000 are injured severely enough to restrict normal activity or require medical attention—a rate of 300 per 1,000 (see Appendix Table 45). Except for infants, accident death rates for children are lower than for adults; nevertheless, accidents are the leading cause of death to children, and the age group under 15 has the highest rate of nonfatal injuries. Children also have the highest rate of bed-disabling injuries. (In this discussion "children" will indicate those under 15 years of age and "infants" those under 1 year of age unless otherwise stated.)

There are currently about 345,000 impairments due to injury in the childhood population. The most frequent types of accidents causing impairments are falls (25 percent) and being struck by a moving object (8 percent). About 11 percent of the children (excluding newborns) discharged from short-stay hospitals during the period July 1957-June 1958 had been hospitalized because of injuries.

Motor-vehicle accidents are the most frequent cause of accidental death in children, at the rate of 8 per 100,000 children. Slightly more than half of these deaths are nonpedestrian. Approximately the same number of children are killed having been hit by cars as die by drowning or in fires or explosions. Other accidental deaths are caused by inhalation and ingestion of food and other objects (2.7 per 100,000), poisoning (1.1), firearms (1.0), and machinery (0.4).

Falls kill about 700 children each year, but they injure over 5,000,000. They are the leading cause of nonfatal injuries to children (90 per every 1,000); next in order are the categories "struck by moving object" (26), "bumped into object or person" (25), and "handled or stepped on rough object" (24). More than a million children are injured annually by animals or insects (19).

Children do not comprise a homogeneous group: changes in growth and development are rapid, as are corresponding changes in accident experience. The infant death rate (from all causes) is especially high.

The same is true of the accident death rate: the rate for infants is 91 per 100,000—nearly three times the rate for children in the age group 1-4 and nearly five times that for the group aged 5-14 (see Appendix Table 1).

Motor vehicles are the greatest single cause of accidental death to children after their first year of life. In the age group 1-4 they cause nearly one-third of all accidental deaths; the rate for this group, 10 per 100,000, is the highest of any childhood age group. From the childhood high of infants, the death rate for nonpedestrian motor-vehicle accidents decreases every year of age through age 4 (see Appendix Table 24); but pedestrian traffic deaths increase in each single year of age (Appendix Table 19).

An important cause of death through age 4 is fire and explosion; the annual rate for this age group is about 7 per 100,000, compared with about 2 for children aged 5-14 (see Appendix Table 31).

Drowning is not a frequent cause of infant death (1.4 per 100,000), but its rate is relatively high in the 1-4 age group (4.2). The rate for age 1 is 6.1, decreasing each year thereafter to 2.7 for age 4. The rate for age group 5-14 is 3.6.

Deaths due to poisoning from solid or liquid substances occur most frequently in the age group 1-4; each year nearly 400 children in this group die from poisoning. Kinds of products involved in poison deaths among different age groups will be discussed in Chapter 4.

Motor vehicles, fires and explosions, and drowning and poisoning together account for about three-fourths of the accidental deaths of children aged 1-4. In addition, nearly 300 children in this age group die each year from falls, 250 from "inhalation and ingestion," and about 80 from firearm accidents.

Children aged 5 and above have the lowest death rate (19 per 100,000) for all accidents in any age group. The motor-vehicle rate is about the same as for the 1-4 group (8); as mentioned earlier, the drowning rate is 3.6. With increasing age there is a decrease of mortality from all sources of poisoning; less than 80 such deaths occur yearly to children aged 5 and over—slightly more than from railway accidents or electric current, and less than from blows by falling or projected objects. The death rate for fire and explosion is also low (2.2 per 100,000), but firearm accidents kill over 400 children in this age group annually.

Death rates for all accidents show a steady decrease from infancy to about age 5; but deaths from different types of accidents show different age distributions. Motor-vehicle pedestrian accidents, for example, increase from a rate of 0.2 per 100,000 for infants to a peak of 6.1 at age 4, decreasing to about 2 after age 10. On the other hand, nonpedestrian motor-vehicle accidents decrease steadily from 7.6 per 100,000 for infants to 3.3 for children 5-9, increasing slightly to 5.4 after age 10. Deaths from falls decrease steadily during the first five years of life from a rate of 5.1 per 100,000 for infants to 0.6 for children 5-14.

Children under six have lower injury rates than do older children in each accident class except home accidents.

Death rates for all accidents are higher among males than among females. In children, however, variation by color is greater, on the average, than variation by sex. Nonwhites generally have higher death rates than do whites, whereas injury rates are higher in whites than in nonwhites—especially for medically attended injuries (see Appendix Table 45). Males have higher injury rates than do females both at home and elsewhere, except for injuries from falls; these occur more frequently to girls than to boys under age ten.

Fire and explosion is the category in which death rates show the greatest color differences. The rate for nonwhite infants is more than seven times as great as that for white infants (see Appendix Table 31). The color ratio narrows slightly after infancy, remaining about five to one until age ten, dropping thereafter to three to one for older children. Except for infants, the drowning rate is higher in white than in nonwhite preschool children (see Appendix Table 33). Death rates for falls among nonwhite children are approximately twice as high as among whites; motor-vehicle pedestrian rates are also somewhat higher among nonwhites, but nonpedestrian rates are lower.

Higher death rates for males than for females is a common epidemiologic finding. In considering accidents, the difference is sometimes attributed to the more active and adventuresome role of males. Some support for this simple supposition is demonstrated by death rates in childhood: the degree of excess of male deaths is lowest in infancy but increases with age. The excesses of male rates are greatest in drowning, where the difference in rates by sex increases with age. Fires and explosions present an exception to this general rule: male deaths slightly outweigh female deaths among infants, but with age the difference becomes smaller. By age three the female rates are substantially higher, and they remain so until about age ten.

The difference between sex variation and color variation in death

rates for children should be noted. When male exceed female accident death rates the excess increases with age, but the excess in nonwhite over white rates tends to decrease with age.

Foreign-born white children under age 5 have twice the death rate of natives for all accidents. The ratio for falls is about 4 to 1, for motor-vehicle accidents (pedestrian and nonpedestrian) and drowning 3 to 1, and for fire and explosion about 2 to 1. Native and foreign-born children age 5-14 have similar rates (see Appendix Table 12).

Nontransport accidents kill over 10,000 children each year and account for approximately two-thirds of all accidental deaths in the age group under 15. Of nontransport accidental deaths that occur in specific places, 71 percent occur in the home (including farm homes) or on the home premises, 6 percent on farms (not including farm homes or their premises), over 3 percent in areas designated for recreation or sport, about 2 percent in residential institutions, and about 1 percent on the street or highway; the remainder occur at such "other specified places" as beaches, lakes, and mountains.

Places of accidental death vary with age, color, and sex; about 93 percent of nontransport deaths of infants in specified places occur in the home, but only about 34 percent to children 10-14 years old occur there. A somewhat greater proportion of nonwhite than white deaths occur in the home (82 percent of the former and 67 of the latter), as do a greater proportion of female than male deaths (83 percent and 63 percent). The difference between the sexes increases with age.

Of 524 children killed each year on farms, over 80 percent are males. About 8 percent of accidental deaths of white children in specified places happen on the farm, as do 3 percent of such nonwhite deaths.

Differences in location can also be classified by type of accident and age. Falls occurring elsewhere than in the home are not frequent in children of preschool age. Over 90 percent of deaths from fire and explosion for each age group occur at home. Ninety-one percent of all infant drownings occur in the home. Most deaths in places of recreation or sport happen to males.

More nonfatal accidental injuries to children occur in the home than anywhere else, according to the National Health Survey. Schools are next in rank, followed by streets and highways; lowest, as might be expected, are industrial sites. Nearly half of all injuries incurred in the home happen to children.

Age-adjusted accident death rates for children are highest in the Mountain, East South Central, and South Atlantic geographic divi-

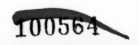

sions of the country and lowest in the Middle Atlantic and New England area. In general, the geographic pattern is similar to that discussed in the section of Chapter 5 entitled "Geography."

The death rate for all accidents is higher among children in non-metropolitan than in metropolitan counties. Nonpedestrian motor-vehicle accident rates for nonmetropolitan counties are nearly twice as high as those for metropolitan counties. The rates for falls, however, are higher in metropolitan counties. Rates are higher for all accidents in metropolitan counties with a central city than in those with no central city.

Data are not available for children under 15, but children under 17 who live on farms have much lower injury rates than those who live either in rural nonfarm or in urban areas.

The outstanding characteristic of monthly accident death rates for the 5-14 age group is the peak reached during the summer months. A lesser but still significant rise during this period is apparent for children under 5. The May-August peak for the 5-14 group coincides, of course, with the period during which children are out of school and engaged in a range of activities within all kinds of environments containing accident potentials.

From the National Health Survey and hospital reporting it can be noted that skull fracture is the outstanding serious injury to children; but data are not available regarding the nature of the outstanding injury causing death. The rate for fractures other than skull fractures is lower in children than among other persons, but lacerations and abrasions are more common among children.

Some types of accidents are almost entirely confined to children: those involving bicycles and washing-machine wringers, for example. Burns—caused by pulling a hot object down upon oneself—poisoning, and drowning in small bodies of water are also problems peculiar to childhood. These are discussed in Chapter 4.

The income-education pattern of injuries to children is discussed below in the section of this chapter entitled "Socioeconomic Factors." One important indication of this pattern is that injuries to children are not a function of low income. Further, observation of the relation between injuries in children and education of family heads shows that the highest rates of injury are in children of college graduates.

It seems reasonable to assume that incidence of accidental injuries to children can be related to social, cultural, and physical environment.

The influence of peers and of parents' cultural patterns, both, must certainly be involved in the frequency and types of such injuries. Stages of growth and development and medical and physical conditions influence accidental injury experience, but the relations are obscure and the literature inconclusive on these matters. Some, nevertheless, are discussed later in this volume.

Since 1900 the trend in accident death rates for children has been downward; but the proportion of childhood deaths due to accidents has increased. For infants, the downward trend in rates is less pronounced and far less regular than for older children. The greatest decreases in rates have occurred in the age group 1-4, the downward trend having been steady in this group since 1910 (see Chart 1.2); but the proportion of all deaths due to accidents for this age group has increased steadily since 1900 and is now triple that of 1930 (Chart 1.1).

The death rate for motor-vehicle accidents to children aged 1-14 has decreased substantially since the 1920's, but this is not true of infant death rates, now considerably higher than they were 35 to 40 years ago. Beginning in 1906-1908, when motor vehicles started coming into use, death rates of children in the 1-14 group began a steep climb. Then, from a peak between 1925 and 1930, they began to fall gradually, the 5-14 rates faster than the 1-4. In the last several years there have been increases from the low rate for children 5-14 (1961) and for children 1-4 (1962). But rates for infants are quite different: a slow, irregular climb to the early 1950's was followed by a slight decrease—but not enough of one to bring the rates to below the 1930 level.

Accidents to the aged. Over 25,000 people 65 years of age or older die from accidental injuries in the United States each year. Approximately 1 of every 1,000 persons aged 65-74, 2 of every 1,000 aged 75-84, and 6 of every 1,000 aged 85 and over die each year from accidents (see Appendix Table 1). "Aged" persons—defined in this discussion as those who are 65 or older—incur three-quarters of all fatal falls, almost one-third of all motor vehicle pedestrian deaths, and over one-quarter of all deaths from "fires and explosions." These three types of accidents account for about 72 percent of all accidental deaths to the elderly.

Approximately 3,000,000 aged persons (a rate of 190 per 1,000) are injured annually (see Appendix Table 45). In general, injury rates are lower in the aged than in younger persons.

Injuries to the elderly result in approximately 100,000,000 days of restricted activity each year, of which over 20,000,000 are bed-days. Approximately 800,000 of those injured in accidents during the year become bed-disabled, and about 200,000 are hospitalized. It is estimated that elderly persons spend approximately 4,000,000 hospital bed days per year for the treatment of injuries (National Health Survey). The greater severity of injuries incurred by the aged than by younger persons is apparent in these high rates.

The average annual number of restricted-activity days among males rises from 4,105 days per 1,000 population (17.4 days per injured person) for the age group 45-64 to 7,458 (41.0 days per person) for those 75 and older. Among females there is a similar rise, from 3,897 (19.3 days per injured person) to 7,707 (36.3 days). Bed-disability days increase from 1,014 per 1,000 population in males aged 45-64 (4.3 days per injured person) to 1,954 per 1,000 in males 75 and over (10.7 days). The increase among females is also great—from 965 (4.8 days) to 2,305 (10.9 days)—and in older groups female rates are higher than male. High rates of bed-disability are associated with retirement, which in turn is associated with age.

It is estimated that there are 1,700,000 persons 65 and older in the noninstitutionalized population of the United States with visual impairments; 142,000 (8.5 percent) of these impairments were caused by injury—a rate of 9.3 per 1,000 persons.

More than one-half of all accidental deaths to the aged are the result of falls, more of which happen to women than to men. Both actual numbers and rates are higher for females. At least 6 of every 1,000 (white) females aged 85 or over who are alive at the beginning of a year will be killed by falls during the year.

Falls account for almost half of the injuries sustained by the elderly, or approximately 1.4 million injuries annually. Sixty-four percent of injuries inside the home and 55 percent of those on exterior home premises are due to falls. It is estimated that a million elderly persons are injured by falls in the home each year.

Of approximately 2,000 accidental injuries among the aged that were reported in one study to the Division of Accident Prevention from hospitals in four areas, about half were due to falls—40 percent or so in males and about 70 percent in females. The proportion of injuries from falls increases with age, reaching about 60 percent of all injuries to males and 80 percent to females in the age 80 and over bracket. At ages over 70, the actual numbers as well as the proportions are higher in women than in men.

Most injuries to older persons from falls occur at home or on the home premises; a higher proportion happen to females (77 percent) than to males (57 percent). For women, the proportion that occur at home increases with age, reaching almost 90 percent at age 80 and over; the pattern in males is not consistent. The highest proportion of home accidents is in the age group over 80, but between 70 and 80 the proportion occurring on the street or highway is high. For older persons, the "resident institution" becomes prominent as a place where accidents occur. About 5 percent of fall injuries among elderly persons occur in resident institutions.

Division of Accident Prevention studies show that fractures are the most common injury resulting from falls among the elderly. Females experience more of these fractures than do males; but the percentage of fractures due to falls increases progressively with age for both sexes. Females suffer more fractured hips from falls than do males, and rates increase as age advances. In fact, "reduction of fractures"—mainly of the hip and pelvis—is the most common surgery among women aged 75 and over. In women 85 and over, hip fractures constitute 30 percent of all injuries due to falls and 56 percent of fractures due to falls.

In cooperation with a county health department, the Division of Accident Prevention of the Public Health Service recently carried out an epidemiologic study of falls among elderly persons in a northeastern city. In interviews, these persons ascribed most fracture cases that did not involve their hips to "slips" and "trips." On the other hand, most of them attributed hip fractures to "weakness" or "spells." About 13 percent blamed loss of balance for their fractures. (The phenomenon of fractured hips in the elderly, and the possible role of bone conditions in this phenomenon, is discussed in the section "Falls," Chapter 4.) Only 7 percent of those injured in falls lived at home with their spouses; almost one-half lived alone. The problems inherent in post-hospital care are obvious.

Death rates from motor-vehicle accidents to pedestrians are extremely high in elderly persons, especially males. Males aged 65 and over constitute only 4 percent of the population, but among them are almost a quarter of the pedestrian deaths. Several reasons including the following three, have been advanced for these exceedingly high rates. (1) Attitude: A large proportion of elderly pedestrians killed are city residents. Their lack of understanding of current traffic characteristics, along with certain fixed ideas, fosters belief in a sort of inherent right to cross the street at will; it must be remembered that their attitudes and habits were, to a large extent, formulated in the horse-drawn era. Many are of lower than average socioeconomic status; many have never driven cars and consequently have only limited understanding of the problems pedestrians present to the driver. Many do not observe traffic lights, nor do they understand the full significance of such signals. (2) Physical conditions: Declining vision and alertness become more of a problem with advancing age—especially during the hours of dusk and darkness, when most fatalities occur. Moreover, the slow pace of the elderly sometimes prevents their making complete street crossings with the control signals, particularly when they leave the curb on a green signal without knowing how long it has been green. Their slow pace also makes it difficult for the motorist to judge position relative to his speed. (3) Unpredictability: Pedestrian actions in general are said to be less predictable than those of drivers; how much more so must this be with the elderly pedestrian! Unpredictability can also be associated with the attitude of the pedestrian that he is "outside the law" in traffic matters.[1]

A brighter side of the picture is the reduction in the pedestrian death rate in recent years: since 1940 the rate among the aged has been cut approximately in half. The reduction in the male rate in recent years has been greater than in the female and greatest in the white male. Nevertheless, the adjusted death rate for males aged 65 and over is still three times as high as that for females, and the elderly male remains a major problem in the achievement of pedestrian safety (see Appendix Table 19).

Nonpedestrian motor-vehicle death rates are high in elderly men. Chart 3.4 shows the death rate for white native-born males for collisions and for the category "run-off-roadway." A fact of great significance is that mortality involving collisions is highest in men over 75: inability to cope with driving conditions, low resistance to injury after a collision, and a higher fatality rate after injury than among younger persons are involved.

Factors contributing to accidents among elderly drivers are inattention, inability to handle certain driving situations, and poor judgment. Some of the more serious faults of older drivers are: failure to yield right-of-way, possibly because of stubbornness or unfamiliarity with the rules of the road; speed, although this factor declines with age—this is a significant cause of accidents among elderly drivers because they drive too fast (or, sometimes, too slowly) for conditions

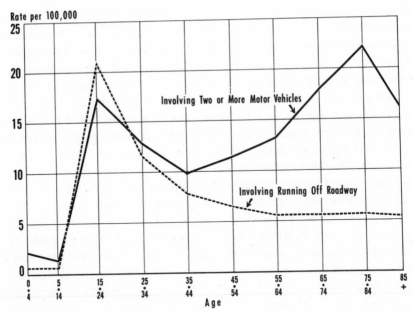

Chart 3.4. Death rates for motor-vehicle accidents to native-born white males by age: United States, 1959-1961.

more often than because they exceed the posted speed limit; improper turning, frequently into the wrong lane; and disregard for signals—a factor that increases with age.

Death rates from fires and explosions are highest in the very young and the very old; they are much higher for males than for females and extremely high for nonwhite persons of both sexes. The rate for nonwhite males aged 65 and over is more than three times as great as for white males, and in women it is approximately five times as great. About three-quarters of these deaths among the elderly occur at home (see Appendix Table 31). Fires and explosions are more important as causes of death than of nonfatal injuries to the aged.

Elderly males have higher accident death rates than do females except at age 85 and over; this late change is due to the higher rate in females from falls. There is a continuous decline in the ratio of male to female deaths from falls in the later years, in contrast to the ratio for motor-vehicle deaths.

In general, the death rate from accidental injuries is higher in nonwhite males than in white persons of either sex; this is so until the later years. In the age groups after 75 changes occur: white rates are higher than nonwhite, and the difference widens with age (see Appendix Table 1). This change in prominence from nonwhite to white and male to female must be studied in relation to type of accident (see Appendix Table 1).

After age 65 the white death rate for falls exceeds the nonwhite, the ratio increasing with age; at 85 and over the white rate is about four times as high as the nonwhite. Moreover, by age 75 the white female rate exceeds the white male rate, and the nonwhite female rate exceeds that of the nonwhite male. (Appendix Table 27 and Chart 3.5 compare these rates at all ages.)

Injury rates are higher for females than for males among the elderly—particularly rates for injuries incurred in the home and on the home premises—largely because of falls. When all injuries are considered, males 65 and over have rates lower than those of younger males. Aged females have higher rates than do either young adult females or aged males.

The higher rates in females hold for injuries involving hospitalization. In the age group 65-74, the female rate for hospitalized injuries (22.9 per 1,000) is about six times that for males (3.7), and for ages 75 and over it is more than twice as high (18.8 versus 8.3).

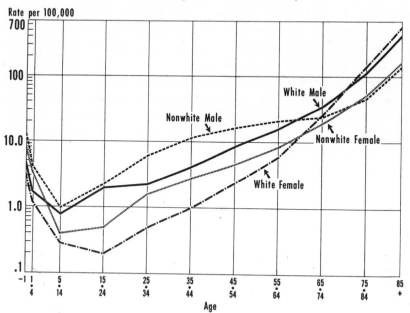

Chart 3.5. Death rates for accidental falls by age, color, and sex: United States, 1959-1961.

The Division of Accident Prevention of the Public Health Service has injury reports from four different areas on accidental injuries to the elderly that are treated in hospitals. These reports show a decrease with age in the number of injuries, and an increase in the ratio of female to male injuries greater than could be accounted for by population differences. Slightly more males than females in the age group 65-69 are treated for accidental injuries; but the figure changes to twice as many females as males in their eighties. The change in ratio is, again, due to the excess of falls in elderly females: injuries from motor vehicles, machinery, blows, fires, and animals are generally higher in males than in females at all ages. Burns from hot substances, however, are more frequent for females in all age groups over 65.

The home is the most common place for injuries and deaths from nontransport accidents to the aged: falls are largely responsible, accounting for about two-thirds of the injuries in the home and over one-half of those on the exterior home premises. Burns and other injuries from fire and explosion are also an important part of the death and injury problem. And of course the street is a continuous hazard from motor vehicles, especially for the elderly male.

In recent years the resident institution, particularly the nursing home and the "home for the aged," has become a common site for accidental injuries. In a special study of a group of nursing homes, the Division of Accident Prevention found that falls were the predominant type of accident, accounting for over 80 percent of all injuries; about one-third of them occurred while getting into or getting up from a bed, wheelchair, commode, or chair. Fractures of the hip and upper leg were common, again emphasizing this problem in the aged.

Insufficient study has been made of the effect of diminished senses (hearing and smell, for example), the ability of the older person to perceive hazards, and the effect of hypertension or other reasons for temporary loss of balance. The possible effect of physical conditions on falls is discussed in the section "Falls," Chapter 4.

Sex

Death rates from accidents are higher in the male than in the female— by approximately 2 to 1 (see Appendix Table 1). The ratio of male to female injury rates does not show as great a difference and is in the order of 1.4 to 1 (see Appendix Table 45). As has been pointed out, when age and type of accident are considered there are substantial differences by sex.

The ratio of male to female death rates for infants is almost 1 to 1, and it increases with age to the middle twenties. In children of school age it is approximately 2 to 1, and in the age group 15-24 approximately 5 to 1. It then decreases with age until, in the age group 85 and over, it is higher for females than for males. This latter shift is—again—reflective of the higher death rate for falls in elderly females.

For injury rates, the male to female ratio is approximately 1 to 1 in the preschool child; it then rises, until in the age group 17-24 the ratio of male to female is about 2.5 to 1. Then it decreases with age until, among the aged, it favors females. This reversal is in large part due to the higher injury rate in the home for aged women; again, of course, the higher rate of injuries from falls is relevant.

The pattern for injuries from falls is similar to that for deaths from falls: the male rate is higher than the female through middle age and the female higher than the male in the later years of life (it is twice the male rate in the group 65 and over). The higher injury rate for falls in female children under 5 is also noteworthy, and was mentioned earlier in the section "Childhood Accidents."

The male death rate for motor-vehicle accidents to pedestrians is higher than the female rate in all age groups and among whites and nonwhites. The same is true of nonpedestrian motor-vehicle accidents. The estimated injury rates from moving motor vehicles (data are not available to distinguish pedestrians from nonpedestrians) are higher for males than for females at all ages up to 65; then, the female rate is higher than the male. (There are few figures for persons in this age group in the National Health Survey sample, however, so that this difference among the aged may not be significant.)

Deaths from fires and explosions are also higher in the male than in the female except in children, where the female rate is higher. Of course, deaths from such accident types as drowning, firearms, electric current, water transport, and machinery are much higher in the male than in the female; and such injury rates as those for machinery, having been struck by a moving object, and lifting and exertion are higher among males. But the injuries classified as "contact with hot object or open flame" are somewhat higher among females (National Health Survey).

Ratios of male to female accident death and injury rates vary with place of occurrence: male ratios, for example, are higher for accidents at work and for accidents occurring in moving motor vehicles. On the other hand, females have a higher injury rate for home accidents.

Race, color, place of birth

In general, nonwhites have a higher death rate from accidental injuries than do whites (see Appendix Table 10); but the injury rate as determined by the National Health Survey is higher for whites (see Appendix Table 45). This higher recorded injury rate in white persons applies to medically attended injuries and activity-restricting injuries; but the rate for bed-disabling injuries and hospitalized injuries is higher among nonwhites. The number of bed-disability days per 1,000 population is also higher for nonwhites, especially for work accidents (see Appendix Table 47). Socioeconomic status, culture (including patterns of use of medical facilities), and the nature of work performed may influence these recorded rates.

Differences in death rates between whites and nonwhites vary by type of accident. Rates are higher among nonwhites for motor-vehicle accidents to pedestrians, fire and explosion, and drowning. Rates are higher for whites for nonpedestrian motor-vehicle accidents, falls, and accidents with machinery, aircraft, and electric current (see Appendix Table 10). Differences between white and nonwhite rates are in part affected by age: in the case of falls, for example, deaths for younger persons are higher in nonwhites, but for old persons they are higher in whites. Age and sex are important considerations in statistical differences between whites and nonwhites.

The death rate for falls is higher in white persons than in any nonwhite group. (This phenomenon is discussed above in "Accidents to the Aged" and below in "Falls," in Chapter 4.) The cause of this is probably the high death rate from falls among elderly white women.

The death rate from fire and explosion is particularly high in non-whites in this country, especially in the South. In fact, the fire and explosion death rate in the United States is one of the highest in the world—chiefly because of the high nonwhite rate.

When class of accident is considered as well as sex, the injury rate for the white male is somewhat higher than for the nonwhite male; this excess is due in large measure to the higher injury rate for accidents in the home among white males. The motor-vehicle injury rate, however, is higher for the nonwhite than the white male. In females, injury rates for moving motor vehicles and for accidents in the home are higher in whites than in nonwhites (see Appendix Table 54).

Among nonwhite persons, Indians have the highest death rate from accidental injuries and Negroes the second. Japanese and Chinese have the lowest rates among those recorded (see Appendix Table 13).

Indians have extremely high death rates from motor-vehicle accidents, both to pedestrians and nonpedestrians, and from drowning; the death rate for firearms is not nearly as high as for drowning, but it is still greater than that of any of the other race-color groups.

Accidents are the second leading cause of death to Indians, whereas they are the fourth leading cause of death to *all* persons in the United States. Accidents are responsible for about 17 percent of deaths among Indians as compared to 6 percent of all deaths in the United States.[2]

The accident death rate for foreign-born white people is almost twice that of native-born whites. Although the former comprise about 5 percent of the population, they sustain about 8 percent of the accidental deaths (see Appendix Table 12). When age is considered, somewhat similar patterns of differences are seen among children and among the elderly; for adults between the ages of 15 and 65, however, there are few rate differences between the native-born and the foreign-born. The median age of the foreign-born is 58 and of the native-born 29, which causes gross differences in unadjusted death rates.

When specific types of accidents are considered, it is observed that deaths from motor-vehicle traffic accidents to pedestrians are about three times as high for the foreign-born white as for the native-born white. Again, these differences are greatest in children under 5 and in the elderly, although there is no age group in which mortality to pedestrians is not greater in the foreign-born than in the native-born. For nonpedestrian deaths the situation is reversed and, except for the age group under 5, native-born whites have higher death rates than foreign-born whites. The death rate from nonpedestrian motor-vehicle accidents to children under 5 is almost three times as great in the foreign-born white as in the native-born white.

For falls, the death rate is much higher in foreign-born than native-born whites in every age group, but particularly in children under 5. Deaths from fire and explosion are greater in the foreign-born than in the native-born white, but again age must be taken into account: the rate is greater for the foreign-born in children under 5, but in all other age groups differences are small and the rate is usually higher in the native-born. The death rate from drowning is somewhat higher in the foreign-born than in the native-born white, and again in children under 5 the differences are greatest.

When country of birth is considered, the highest death rate for accidents is found among the Irish, Swedish, and Norwegians; low rates are found among those born in Italy, the United Kingdom, Poland, Russia, Hungary, and Czechoslovakia. The highest death rate from motor-vehicle accidents is for Mexicans; Swedes and Norwegians are next. Low rates are noted for persons from Italy, the United Kingdom, Germany, and Poland. The death rate for non-motor-vehicle accidents is higher for every other country of birth than for the United States. Moreover, the death rate (motor-vehicle and non-motor-vehicle, both) in the United States for a person of foreign birth is even greater than the corresponding rate in his "home country." This is evident in Table 3.1, which shows the crude death rates for these types of accidents among the foreign-born in the United States as compared with the rates for residents in their countries of origin. These comparisons are informative; but allowance is not made for differences in age distribution of the populations, and there are also variations in methods of recording basic data. In no instance is the ratio of total United States deaths to total native deaths less than 1. The ratio varies from 5 to 1 for Ireland to 1.4 to 1 for Germany. For motor-vehicle accidents the ratio of Mexicans in the United States to native Mexicans is 17 to 1. For non-motor-vehicle accidents, the ratio for Ireland is 6 to 1; Mexico has the lowest ratio—1.2 to 1.

It is interesting to speculate on reasons for the comparatively high accident death rate of foreign-born persons in the United States. Besides differences in age distribution, role change, change of culture, and what might be called "incomplete social integration" are, doubtless, factors in this high death rate.

Marital status

As is true for most causes of death, death rates for accidents are lower at all ages in married persons than in single, surviving, or divorced persons. It has frequently been pointed out that the death rate is highest for widows and widowers, followed by divorced and then single persons. This phenomenon is discussed by Mindel Sheps,[3] who also mentions the possibility of errors in census figures and in classification of death certificates. Joseph Berkson[4] discusses the fact that almost all causes of death show similar differential rates when classed by marital status and considers the incredibility of such a circumstance. He points out that death rates "increase monotonically in the order, married, single, divorced, etc.," and he points out that one must not be guilty of the "fallacy of misplaced concreteness." But Albert Iskrant[5] states that "it can be said that these mortality data are not in

Table 3.1 Ratio of crude death rates: foreign-born residents of the United States to residents of countries of birth, 1959-61

| | Crude death rate | | | | | | | | |
| | Foreign born in the United States U.S. death rate | | | Residents in country of birth Native death rate | | | Ratio: U.S. foreign born to residents of country of birth | | |
Country	Total (E800-E962)	Motor-vehicle (E810-E835)	Non-motor-vehicle (E800-E802, E840-E962)	Total (E800-E962)	Motor-vehicle (E810-E835)	Non-motor-vehicle (E800-E802, E840-E962)	Total (E800-E962)	Motor-vehicle (E810-E835)	Non-motor-vehicle (E800-E802, E840-E962)
Ireland[c]	157.2	28.4	128.8	32.1	10.2	21.9	4.9	2.8	5.9
Sweden[b]	154.0	31.4	122.6	46.4	14.6	31.8	3.3	2.2	3.9
Norway[b]	147.6	36.9	110.7	43.7	8.4	35.3	3.4	4.4	3.1
Denmark[b]	114.9	28.6	86.3	44.8	16.9	27.9	2.6	1.7	3.1
Austria[c]	102.5	27.5	75.0	65.6	22.2	43.4	1.6	1.2	1.7
Mexico[a]	98.0	51.7	46.3	41.9	3.0	38.9	2.3	17.2	1.2
Canada[a]	89.0	28.4	60.6	52.7	21.2	31.5	1.7	1.3	1.9
Czechoslovakia[b]	78.8	21.2	57.6	–	13.4	–	–	1.6	–
Germany[c],[d]	78.7	20.6	58.1	57.8	25.6	32.2	1.4	0.8	1.8
Hungary[c]	77.7	25.5	52.2	34.9	6.9	28.0	2.2	3.7	1.9
Poland[b]	77.4	20.6	56.8	33.4	4.5	28.9	2.3	4.6	2.0
Italy[b]	68.1	18.9	49.2	40.9	17.8	23.1	1.7	1.1	2.1

Source: Demographic Yearbook, 1962 (United Nations: New York, 1962), tables 4 and 5, and Epidemiological and Vital Statistics Report (World Health Organization: Geneva, 1965), 18:117-124.

a. Crude death rate for residents in country of birth, 1959.
b. Crude death rate for residents in country of birth, 1960.
c. Crude death rate for residents in country of birth, 1961.
d. Federal Republic of Germany.

conflict with hypotheses of accident causation which stress the emotional or behavioral aspects." Perhaps it is in the exception to Berkson's "monotonic order" that the clues to the causation of accidents and their association with social and psychological factors are seen.

Appendix Table 2 shows the death rate for all accidents by age, color, sex, and marital status. After age 19, the rates for married persons are always the lowest. The rates for widows and widowers are higher than those of the divorced up to about age 40, when rates of the divorced become greater than those of survivors. At about age 65, the rate for widows and widowers becomes lower than the rate for the single and stays that way for older groups. This tendency is more pronounced in females than in males, and may be related to the fact that, among the elderly, women more often survive their husbands than men do their wives. Age-adjusted rates by marital status and type of accident are shown in Appendix Table 14; the same general patterns are evident. Motor-vehicle accidents to pedestrians, falls, fires, drownings—all seem to follow somewhat similar patterns.

Elderly married persons (with the exception of occupants of motor vehicles) have the lowest death rates from the leading types of accidents of any marital status group. The age-adjusted death rate for motor-vehicle accidents to nonpedestrians is higher for widows and widowers than for any other group. This pattern, true in all younger age groups also, raises questions about the classification of marital status when both husband and wife are killed in the same automobile accident: if one dies some hours or so before the other, is the person who died later specified on the death certificate as married or as a widow or widower? The higher death rate for widows and widowers than for married persons from motor-vehicle accidents would be accounted for in large part if the latter classification were always selected.

Another phenomenon worth noting is the higher death rate among married than among single young persons under 20 from motor-vehicle accidents to nonpedestrians (see Appendix Table 25). This is particularly clear in the white male, so that the question of a departure from "normality" is again raised: females usually marry at a younger age than do males, and it is possible that males who marry in their teens are not conforming to current social patterns—a characteristic that could be in some way related to their greater likelihood of death in motor-vehicle accidents. There is also a tendency among married white persons under 25 toward a higher death rate from fires than among unmarried white persons: this may indicate that young married whites are inclined to live in housing with more fire hazards. Another item of interest is the high death rate for nonpedestrian motor-vehicle accidents to married white females in their later years; although it is impossible from the data available to distinguish between the driver and passengers of the car, it may perhaps be assumed that the elderly white married female is exposed to a higher risk of death in a motor-vehicle accident because she drives with her husband.

Injury rates by marital status show less variation between groups than do death rates (see Appendix Table 55). Here the marital status of people in the numerator is the same as that of those in the denominator because the information is obtained through home interviews. Therefore, whatever variations do exist probably reflect a variety of actual experience rather than "quirks" in the denominator. Married people again have lower injury rates for all types of accidents than do the "never-married" (single); but the "other" group (divorced and separated) also has generally lower rates than those of the single. It should be pointed out that variation by marital status seems to be greater for males than for females.

In injury rates by marital status, there is variation by class of accident. For moving motor-vehicle injuries to males, the "never-married" have a much higher rate than the married or the "other" group (see Appendix Table 55). For accidents while at work, however, never-married men have the lowest accidental injury rate. For "other places," which includes public places, the never-married have by far the highest injury rate among males. For females, there is little difference in the moving motor-vehicle injury rates between the never-married and the married. For accidental injuries at home, however, the married rate is higher than that of the never-married, and the rate among the "other" group is highest. Married women have the lowest rate of accidents at work.

Data are not available for groupings by sex, age, and type of accident; but within the total category of accidental injuries and without consideration of sex, it appears that with advancing age rates tend to be lowest among the never-married (see Appendix Table 49).

Socioeconomic factors

In the opening paragraph of the present volume we quoted from Abel Wolman regarding the effect of mores and practices on injury rates and other health problems.[6] The structure of our society, with its great variety of cultural elements, influences the values and behavior of different groups and their reactions to specific situations, thus affecting their accident involvement. Considering this, social and cultural factors are perhaps best viewed as part of the chain of causation in terms of their effect on over-all accident probability, as well as their influence on other factors still—factors that are involved more directly in the accident situation. Cultural factors influence economic factors and in turn are influenced by economic factors.

It is our belief that the social and cultural elements influencing the occurrence of accidental injuries are a group product and therefore are amenable to change by organized effort. The group approach may contribute more to accident prevention than attempts to change individual behavior ever could.

The influences of income and education and such social forces as peer relationships, customs, and mores will be discussed here. It should be emphasized again that no one factor causes an accident, but that various factors contribute to its probability and increase the likelihood and severity of injury. Of course these factors are not independent, and frequently they are interrelated to a large degree. Some factors will be discussed separately and others will be summarized in groups. Items included will be income, education, occupation, housing, living arrangements, family (including its supervision), peer group, major life disruptions (including involvement, attitudes [group], customs, and values), and alcohol.

A belief held widely is that the lower the income and the economic status of a person or family, the higher the accidental injury rate. Data from the National Health Survey and elsewhere do not support this view. The injury rate is lowest in families with annual incomes of under $2,000 (see Appendix Table 45), as is the rate for medically attended injuries—but not for activity-restricting injuries. It is possible, of course, that persons of very low income do not seek the medical attention for injuries that those of higher economic status do. The fact that activity-restricting injuries for ages 15-64 are lowest in persons in the high income group brings to mind the possibility that persons in families earning $7,000 and more annually are engaged in occupations where an injury would not be as likely to cause restriction of activity (see Appendix Table 50). Another pertinent observation, with regard to accident class, is that for moving motor vehicles the highest injury rates are in persons in the upper income groups, whereas injuries at work are lowest in families having an annual income of either under $2,000 or over $7,000. Injuries that occur in the home are least frequent in the lowest income group (see Appendix Table 46).

The lower injury rate among older than among younger age groups may be related to the fact that, in general, older persons are more likely to be in the lower income groups. Thus, the apparent lower injury rates of low income groups may be due to the large proportion of aged among them. Again, too, it is possible that persons in the lower economic groups may not always seek medical care for injuries; on the other hand, if they live near out-patient departments and the custom in the area is to go to such departments with illnesses and injuries, they may be *more* likely to seek medical care than would persons of higher income.

Greater rates of bed-disability in lower than in higher income groups may reflect their large proportion of older persons, as well as the greater tendency of the elderly than of younger persons toward long periods of disability from injuries.

Data from the National Health Survey show that, in general, the variation in the incidence of injury according to the education of the family head follows that according to family income. The incidence rates are higher for males and females in the upper income and education groups, except for the age group 25-44 (see Appendix Table 52). The same pattern is evident with regard to accident class: injuries from moving motor vehicles are highest among the best educated (also those of highest income) and work injuries are lowest.

Other National Health Survey data suggest that most injuries in the labor force are among laborers, craftsmen, and operatives and least among managers and sales people. In the age groups 17-24 and 65 and over, operatives and kindred workers have extremely high rates. High rates in the younger age group may be due to lack of experience and in the older to decreasing physical ability (see Appendix Table 57).

When class of accident is considered it is noted that injuries from moving motor vehicles are higher in operatives and farm laborers than they are in farmers and clerical workers. This may partly explain the high total accidental injury rate for operatives in the young age groups. For work accidents, rates are high among laborers, craftsmen, operatives, farmers, and farm laborers, and, as might be expected, lowest in sales workers, clerical workers, managers, and professional workers. Injuries from home accidents are highest in household workers and among professional and technical people (see Appendix Table 58).

Data for computing valid accident death rates by occupation are not easily obtainable. However, a publication of the Public Health Service for 1950[7] shows that the standardized mortality ratio for accidents at work was highest for laborers, operatives, and farmers and lowest for clerical workers, professionals, and sales workers. Deaths from accidents not incurred at work have the same general pattern.

The literature on accident prevention is replete with statements that home accidents can be associated with poor housing and low socio-economic status; but available data on income and education do not support the accidental injury-low economic status theory. Neverthe-less, there are certain hazards that are clearly associated with poor housing: lead poisoning, falls on rickety stairs, and cuts from trash and broken glass, for example; it would also appear that such injuries as those from washing-machine wringers and fires and explosions could be high. On the other hand, there are types of accidents which would obviously occur more frequently in the higher income groups. Injuries from power mowers, for example, would not be expected to be high in tenement housing. Perhaps the best summation of the situation is that accidental injuries are no respecters of persons or housing, but rather that type of accident varies with social, economic, and cultural patterns.

Living arrangements have some bearing on frequency of injury. In general, people who live alone or with others not related to them have the highest accidental injury rates (see Appendix Table 53). This is the case for all age groups except 45-64, where differences are small. However, because so many "relatives" are children, the rate for persons in the "unmarried" category is highest for all ages. The category "living with relatives—married" has the lowest rates, corresponding to situations already described for married persons in the section "Marital Status."

The same pattern with regard to living arrangements is found in the incidence of injury from motor vehicles. On the other hand, the injury rate from home accidents is highest in persons not married but living with relatives—a situation that doubtless reflects the high home acci-dent rate among children.

Every "group" to which an individual belongs has some influence in developing and modifying his attitudes and beliefs. Interpersonal relations (those between parent and child, for example), many aspects of child rearing, daily routines, and activities are influential in de-termining accident experience. The kind of supervision provided for a child by his parent or another responsible adult certainly is an important underlying factor in many injuries like accidental ingestion of poisonous substances or those incurred by washing-machine wringers.

William Langford's study suggests that "nonaccident parents" are close to their children and supervise them carefully, and that these families have more fun together than "accident families."[8] Backett and Johnston in a study of 101 children injured in pedestrian road accidents compared the children with a nonaccident control group and found—among other things—that maternal preoccupation, lack of protection during play, and fewer play facilities were factors associated with the accidents.[9] Morris Schulzinger suggests that teaching a child safe practices by example and providing him with continuing exposure to a peaceful, orderly home environment may be important aids to "immunizing" him against accidents. He suggests that persons encourage the child toward safe practices and show him by example that they themselves engage in such practices.[10]

It seems likely that the example set by parents in the motor vehicle strongly influences the child's attitude, especially in later life when he himself drives. "Cop-watching," unpleasant remarks about other drivers, and boasts about speed and the breaking of traffic regulations probably profoundly affect attitudes of children—attitudes difficult to change when driving age is reached. This problem is magnified if a child's peers, who in turn are influenced by *their* parents' attitudes, exert similar influences upon him.

The behavior of children and perhaps of older persons is unquestionably influenced by their peers; the risks a child takes are to a large extent determined by the mores and play patterns of his "group." It appears that driving after drinking and "chicken-out" competitions—not only in driving, but in other forms of activity—have a profound influence on the death and injury rate of young people. The progress of program development in accident prevention depends on the extent to which alternative behaviors can be developed in peer groups that will permit the demonstration of new safe behavior patterns. Programs based on efforts to change group behavior through group discussion and other methods offer a profitable line of endeavor toward accident prevention, especially among young people.

Major disruptions, especially in the later years of life, also seem to have a pronounced influence on the incidence of accidental injuries: reduction in income and scale of living, moving to different—sometimes deteriorated—quarters, death of a spouse or loved one, serious illness in self or spouse, and other unfortunate occurrences so common among elderly people. Such changes (which often involve moving to the home of a younger family with different ways of life) can create situations with accident potential, especially when accompanied by psychomotor and sensorimotor decline.

It has been speculated that both "under-involvement" and "over-involvement" in the social environment are associated with high accidental injury rates; this is an area which merits further research. Role changes, many of which are associated with aging, are also believed to affect the incidence of accidents.

It seems reasonable to assume that people's attitudes, whether formed individually or by group, influence frequency of accidental injuries and types of accidents. General attitudes exist, which are determined by "society"; but it is well to remember that there are also cultural subgroups. What may appear deviant to a larger group may represent conformity to a subgroup's cultural norms. Different groups may differ in accident susceptibility because of different norms of risk behavior or safety behavior. The risk behavior of hot-rodders or leather-jacketed motorcycle enthusiasts may be entirely different from the risk behavior of the tennis crowd.

Edward Suchman states that "cultural and social factors are of prime importance in the etiology of accidents—in terms of both frequency and type."[11] This is obviously so in regard to the motor vehicle and other modes of transportation and is probably equally true of guns and sports. Play patterns involving toy guns and other imitations of dangerous instruments, for example, when unaccompanied by an appropriate safety program may influence injury patterns in later life. McFarland and Moore, in *Youth and the Automobile,* point out the cultural implications of the automobile to the hot-rodder and to other young people and describe it as a symbol of power and an outlet for hostility and aggression, discourtesy, emotional conflict, and revolt. They also emphasize the automobile as a status symbol and discuss its effect on the experience of the young during school years.[12]

To a large extent, customs influence attitudes toward the law; in most segments of the population it is quite common to regard traffic-law violations as "folk crimes"—not law violations at all to one's peers.[13] Not considering specific hazards (the automobile, guns, high-diving, and so on), there is in the United States a general cultural acceptance that exposure to risk is associated with manhood and is part of our heritage. Potentially dangerous activities must be accompanied by appropriate safety training so that proper safeguards can be utilized when needed. Persons engaged in promoting measures of accident prevention greatly encourage learn-to-swim, learn-to-ski, learn-to-shoot, and other such programs.

Certain social patterns not only involve but encourage drinking. To the extent that drinking is an accepted practice throughout the country, as is driving or taking part in other hazardous activities after drinking, alcohol is obviously a problem in accident causation; and because social factors influence the patterns of alcohol use in a community, they, too, are involved. One solution to the drinking problem may be that of social control: attempting to change the norms of cultural groupings large or small. To whatever extent such groups can be influenced to exert more caution after drinking, or to moderate the use of alcohol before driving or engaging in other hazardous activities, reduction of injuries may be accomplished.

Psychological factors

There is evidence that personal factors and factors related to attitudes play a role in accident involvement, and that certain psychophysical and sensory variables—reaction time, visual and auditory acuity, depth perception, and so on—may be involved. To date, however, attempts to isolate stable personality traits for the development of a personality profile of the "safe" individual have met with little success. Not enough research has been done to discriminate with accuracy between the accident-susceptible and the nonsusceptible person, although studies have shown that some relationships between them do exist.

There are many difficulties encountered in studying risk-taking, even under laboratory conditions, and translating experimental results into actual situations: for instance, it is not yet clear how closely driving simulators reproduce "on-the-road" experience. Moreover, it is difficult to limit research on psychological variables, to the exclusion of the physical, social, and cultural environments in which people operate. The problem is complicated in that psychological response is not stable and varies according to situation; certain psychological factors that predispose accidents may be of a somewhat temporary nature.

Many attempts have been made to identify the "accident prone," with only minor success. McFarland and others[14] have concluded that accident proneness is a much more restricted phenomenon than it was thought to be originally; they suggest concentration on persons who are "accident-repeaters."

Because of the frightful impact motor-vehicle accidents have made upon the nation, much research has been undertaken to discover whether there are personality traits and psychological factors distinguishing the "good driver" from the "bad driver," and whether it is possible to predict in advance the accident susceptibility of a particular personality. Statistics show that those under 25 and over 65 years of age have disproportionately high death rates from motor-vehicle accidents, but the reasons for this have not yet been identified. There is some indication, evidenced in the studies of McFarland and others mentioned above, that certain stable or enduring characteristics can be associated with high frequency of motor-vehicle accidents: these include youthfulness, low rate of intelligence, and personality composition that features egocentricity, aggressiveness, antisocial feelings, and social irresponsibility.

In a study conducted by Beamish and Malfetti it was determined that adolescent traffic violators differ from adolescent nonviolators with respect to certain psychological characteristics. Significant differences were found in measures of emotional stability, social conformity, objectivity, and mood.[15]

A study by John Conger and others suggests that, in general, the "accident personality" is unconventional and self-oriented; has feelings of dissatisfaction with everyday life; lacks clearly defined goals; is unable to control hostility; tends toward "acting out" behavior either physically or verbally; shows poor judgment; lacks contact with reality, especially in social relationships; may show a psychopathologic tendency toward hostility, withdrawal, or excessive immaturity. This study portrays the accident-repeater as a person who is unable to adjust to stress, whose attempts toward upward mobility are generally thwarted, and who has feelings of insecurity.[16]

Tillmann and Hobbs discuss the high accident record that appears to be associable with aggressiveness and conflict with authority, originating in an insecure home background and continuing in a history of frequent conflict with community standards. Drivers with few accidents are usually "serious, stable, well-adjusted individuals with well-integrated home backgrounds."[17]

Other studies of attitudinal and personality correlates of accident susceptibility suggest such characteristics as egocentricity, impulsiveness, conflict with authority, desire for autonomy, anxiety, pessimism, low morale, fatalism, introversion, and unstable employment records or negative attitudes toward employment.

Many studies purport to have identified abnormal personality traits that are associable with a high incidence of accidents or with particular types of accidents; these traits are frequently only the product of the author's imagination or of his pet beliefs, often existing in everyone if one but looks for them. Characteristics identified through epidemiologic studies should be subjected to the most rigorous tests under controlled conditions. This is being attempted in a current study of 17,000 drivers in Connecticut, conducted jointly by the Division of Accident Prevention and the State of Connecticut. As part of a multiple screening test, an attitude questionnaire has been administered to these drivers; when scored, the results will be related to their subsequent driving experience.

Conclusions from studies by Vita Krall,[18] Lawrence LeShan,[19] and others tend to support the hypothesis that conflict with authority bears a definite relation to accident causation; and such studies as those by Krall, Flanders Dunbar,[20] and Irwin Marcus and others[21] indicate that tension and anxiety may have similar relations. A number of studies suggest some relation between accidents and the unconscious wish for self-injury or self-destruction.

Three abnormal behavior patterns which often occur in normal individuals under "temporary emotional upset" are classified by the American Medical Association Committee on Medical Aspects of Automobile Injuries and Deaths as follows: (1) absorption with a problem to such an extent that the individual is indifferent and inattentive to external conditions; (2) despondence so great as to cause psychomotor retardation; and (3) heightened aggressiveness or impulsiveness to such a degree as to impair judgment and decrease caution.[22]

Physical and medical conditions

Medical conditions and physical defects are frequently associated with accidents in the literature available on the subject. In many instances the association is nebulous, but in others a direct causal relation is established with reasonable certainty. Such variation is to be expected because in this area it is especially difficult to evaluate causal factors. Difficulties can arise because of the many elements involved in accidents; because of failure to diagnose a disease prior to an accident; or because it is frequently impossible to establish a precise association between a medical condition and an accident. Even if a disease state has been diagnosed prior to an accident the etiological relationship may remain obscure.

Through careful investigation of some of the well-defined types of accidents it is possible to identify conditions to which accident causation may be reliably ascribed. Such determinations are made frequently by medical examiners' offices in many areas of the world, unfortunately often without sufficient investigation and therefore occasionally erroneously.

Just as there are difficulties in determining the causal relation between an individual's disease state and his accident, so, too, there are many problems in analyzing the diseases and accidents of an entire population. Some statistical investigations have been made of these relations, however. In the Eastern Health District of Baltimore, a study of white families over a five-year period (1938-1943) showed that "a consistently higher percentage of individuals who had repeated accidents during a specified period had some chronic disease than was true of individuals who had no accidents." Selwyn Collins, the author of the study, concluded that "the presence of chronic disease apparently adds to the liability to accident for the individual afflicted with the disease."[23]

A study of women involved in accidents has revealed an association between accidents and menstruation, suggesting that increased lethargy during menstruation and the premenstruum is responsible for both lowered judgment and slow reaction time.[24]

The Division of Accident Prevention of the Public Health Service studied the records of 13,000 members of a "pre-paid" health group (all care provided or paid for by the organization involved). The study showed that, up to age 40 (data were inconclusive beyond this point), the percentage of accidental injuries treated was higher among members with previously diagnosed medical conditions than among others. Of nine broad groups of medical conditions diagnosed, three showed a relation to incidence of accidental injuries: disease of the nervous system and sense organs (under age 10); allergic, endocrine system, metabolic, and nutritional diseases (under age 30); and disease of the digestive system (older persons). But it was not possible to relate a type of accident to a particular diagnosis, perhaps because of the small number of cases.[25]

Limited statistical evidence is available to show that physical and medical conditions play a more important part in some accidents than in others, and that certain physical and medical conditions predispose certain types of accidental injuries; attempts to relate all accidental injuries to all physical and medical conditions, however, conceal by aggregation a network of more specific associations. For this reason, most reported studies have been directed toward a specific type of accident or injury, a specific population group, or a specific environment.

Much of the research aimed at uncovering the relation of physical or medical conditions to specific types of accidents has been based on experiences with motor vehicles. The purpose of some of these studies has been to identify persons with diseases or impairments that might make them higher-risk drivers or that might cause accidents. As increasingly precise information is gained, programs can be devised to establish policies of driver licensing that are more consistent with recognized problems and that approach a reasonable balance between limitation of the driver's privilege to drive and the welfare of the community. Some physical and medical conditions so interfere with safe driving that studies to establish their relation to accidents are unnecessary; others require individual assessment. Peterson and Petty have studied 192 fatalities in which motor-vehicle accidents were involved. On autopsy, 156 of the 192 deaths were classified as due to accidental trauma; 36 (19 percent) were classified as due to natural causes, all of which were related to the cerebro-cardiovascular system.[26]

The Division of Accident Prevention, in cooperation with the Cuyahoga County (Ohio) Coroner's Office, came to similar conclusions after a study of 225 single motor-vehicle accidents. Of the drivers (all 225) examined at autopsy, 57 deaths were classified as due to natural causes—most related to diseases of the heart.[27] Julian Waller has compared the records of 2,672 California drivers reported to have certain chronic medical conditions and 922 not known to have such conditions, and has found that "drivers with diabetes, epilepsy, cardio-vascular disease, alcoholism and mental illness averaged twice as many accidents per 1 million miles of driving and one and three-tenths to one and eight-tenths times as many violations per 100 thousand miles as drivers in the comparison group on an age-adjusted basis." He points out that this report contains an excess of epilepsy cases due to a compulsory reporting statute, and that it might also reflect irregular reporting of mental illness, alcoholism, drug usage, diabetes, and some chronic diseases; and he cautions that no conclusions can be drawn about the accident experience of those with similar conditions that are not known to the California Department of Motor Vehicles.[28]

Disabled veterans and handicapped persons holding motor-vehicle registrations were studied in Massachusetts. A group numbering 625 was paired with a group of 625 nondisabled drivers and matched according to sex, age, and years of driving experience; the records of accident and nonaccident citations issued to the two groups were then compared. The reliability of the information obtained is limited; the accidents described do not necessarily involve injury; there is ambiguity in the descriptions of offenses for which citations were issued; the comparison is only for operators of passenger vehicles, not commercial vehicles; there is no adequate control on the number of miles driven by each group. Keeping these limitations in mind, it was discovered that the disabled had better driving records than the nondisabled.[29]

Vision and hearing are obviously involved in the operation of motor vehicles. When these functions are below normal, measurement of the degree of impairment and estimation of the increased risk evokes many discussions. There have been studies published on the effects of impaired vision and defective hearing, but the subject is far from closed. A statement addressed to the physician is offered by a committee of the American Medical Association. The committee believes that "patients whose corrected vision, tested under standard conditions, is 20/40 or better may be advised that this vision is adequate for the task of operating a private vehicle. Those with vision less than 20/40 should be referred to an ophthalmologist to ascertain if vision can be improved. Patients with less than 20/70 corrected vision in the better eye should be advised not to drive. At present there is no uniformity of opinion regarding the safe driving ability of individuals with visual acuity between 20/40 and 20/70. Furthermore, there are no scientific data available which permit the establishment of fixed standards."[30]

This committee also suggests that persons with visual form fields of less than 110 degrees should be advised not to drive; visual form fields of 140 degrees or more are considered adequate. Other ophthalmologic pathology, including but not limited to ocular muscle imbalance, color blindness, dark adaptation, and susceptibility to glare, are also discussed in the report. The relation to driving for varying degrees of impairment due to these ocular conditions is still not accurately known.

The effects on driving of disorders of hearing and balance related to otolaryngologic pathology are even less precisely identified than effects of visual disturbances. The American Medical Association guide considers deafness disqualifying for operation of commercial vehicles but not private vehicles. Dizziness, from any cause, is recognized as a much greater potential hazard.

The list of physical conditions and diseases that might have effects on driving under selected circumstances approximates a medical catalogue. Virtually no disease or physical impairment can be totally excluded from possible relation to motor-vehicle accidents.

The relation of physical impairment and disease to causation is not limited to motor-vehicle accidents. When other accidents are examined, the problem is equally complex and even less well documented. In England, of 209 adults receiving in-patient care for burns and scalds in a particular hospital area, 35 (17 percent) were diagnosed as epileptics.[31] An insurance company has found that dizzy spells, epileptic seizures, and other illnesses were reported as possible contributory factors in the cases of approximately one-fourth of 181 adult policyholders who died in falls from windows.[32]

The Division of Accident Prevention has initiated investigations into the relation between osteoporosis and fractures in the elderly. Falls involving fractured hips have been most common in elderly white females, the group hypothesized to have the highest prevalence of osteoporosis. J. H. Sheldon has suggested that a defect in the central nervous-system control of posture and gait may be responsible for many unexplained falls in the aged.[33]

A study comparing secondary causes specified on certificates of death from accidents in the home with secondary causes on certificates of death from cancer concludes that "chronic illness, per se, is more frequently encountered among persons dying of home accidents than among those dying of cancer." The authors of this study, conducted in New York, caution that mortality statistics on elderly people may reflect their inability to recover from home accidents rather than an actual increased incidence of injuries.[34]

Temporary conditions

There are many conditions other than actual disease states that may impair a person's performance and contribute to his accidental injury. Although the actual acute state of certain disabling diseases may indeed be "temporary," the subject matter of this section is not these diseases but essentially nonanatomical conditions that may significantly impair a person's ability to perform complex tasks.

Of these conditions alcohol receives the most publicity, and it has been the subject of a great amount of research—appropriately so because of its frequent involvement in accident causation. Investigation of the role played by alcohol in the reduction of man's performance has, however, been based mostly on driving experiences. The relation between alcohol and nontransport accidents has received far less attention, although it is known that the two are very closely connected.

Drugs are taken frequently by great numbers of persons before and during the performance of complex tasks. Some drugs are known to have the side effect of inducing drowsiness, but others are less well defined. Unexpected primary or secondary effects can contribute to accidental injury. Thus, the loss of attention and concern brought on by some hypnotics—including sedatives, soporifics, ataraxics, tranquilizers, antiepileptics, barbiturates, and bromides—may constitute a definite hazard while driving or performing other complex tasks. Similarly, sleep induced rapidly or to unexpected depths may contribute to the death of smokers in bed or in overstuffed furniture. To the problem of prescribed drugs must be added the more common "over-the-counter" drugs.

The exact relation of most drugs to the performance of various complex tasks is not well known; and complications arise with the rapid production of new drugs. The difficulty of designing methods for chemical analysis of the blood of accident victims makes diagnosis difficult or impossible. Even when such methods have been devised there will be, for some time, a lack of comparative data upon which to judge the effect of various concentrations of a drug. Nevertheless, reasonable public health measures need not await conclusive data. Physicians can advise patients who take certain medications about their possible effects on driving or other tasks. If informed on the subject, the general public can also take reasonable precautions.

Less dramatic than drugs are temporary states like common fatigue, inattentiveness, transient distractions, and the elusive but intriguing concept of "road hypnosis." This latter condition may be a combination of the fatigue-inattentiveness factor and the influence of the monotonous rhythms of mechanical tasks. The concept fascinates many but has been adequately investigated and described by few.

Temporary emotional disturbances may contribute to inattentiveness or poor judgment, thereby causing accidental injury. To date such factors constitute an essentially unknown quantity of accident causation, although it seems probable that significant emotional disturbances could so interfere with performance that accidents result. Precise description of environmental factors and of the emotional disturbance and the characteristics of the victim prior to the accident must await adequate research.

4 / AGENT OR TYPE OF ACCIDENT

The large number of agents involved in accidental injury causation are difficult to discuss without referring to specific types of accidents in particular circumstances. Sometimes the agent of the accident (a loose rug that is tripped on, for example) is different from the agent of the injury (the desk or fireplace struck); sometimes they are the same, as when a knife slips. Because the variety of possible agents is bewildering, this presentation will be simplified by discussing type of accident (fall, machinery) with occasional reference to specific agent (hole in sidewalk, power saw). To the extent possible the discussion will also refer to the interaction of accident and agent with host and environment.

Railway accidents
The International Code gives priority to motor vehicles over railways, so that a collision between a motor vehicle and a train is considered a motor-vehicle accident. The death rate in the United States is about 0.7 per 100,000 persons for motor-vehicle and train collisions (see Appendix Table 10).

There are about 1,000 deaths each year from railway accidents not including collisions with motor vehicles—a rate of 0.6 per 100,000. The rate is very low for the age groups under 15 (0.0 or 0.1); it increases gradually to 1.0 for the group 45-74 and then to 1.8 for ages 85 and over. In general, the male rate is about ten times that of the female, and the nonwhite twice that of the white (see Appendix Table 10). Railway accidents are most frequent during the summer months, but the reverse is true of collisions of trains with motor vehicles (see Appendix Table 15). The death rate for railway accidents decreased gradually from 3.4 per 100,000 in 1930 to 0.5 in 1963.

The Interstate Commerce Commission publishes data concerning injuries and deaths on railroads. The Commission's publication indicates that the number of persons killed per 1,000,000 train-miles increased from 3.4 in 1955 to 4.1 in 1964. Nearly 60 percent of the total railway deaths in 1962 were from grade-crossing accidents, although only 13 percent of the injuries were incurred in such accidents. There were about 27,000 injuries altogether during 1962 from railway accidents. In that year, 27 passengers, 604 trespassers, and 142 employees were killed in train and train-service accidents; injuries were to 2,109 passengers, 595 trespassers, and 11,374 employees.[1]

Motor-vehicle accidents

Deaths and injuries from motor vehicles happen in a variety of ways to a variety of people. The victims may be drivers and passengers of cars or they may be pedestrians, including bystanders. Some deaths and many injuries occur in motor vehicles that are not moving: people are killed or seriously injured by cars falling off jacks, for example; children especially suffer many injuries from slammed doors, bumped heads, and other such accidents. According to the National Health Survey, estimated annual injuries from nonmoving motor vehicles number about 2,000,000. Deaths and injuries occur, too, in moving motor vehicles that are not in traffic. The figures presented hereafter will refer to moving motor vehicles, and the discussion will be limited in general to traffic accidents.

Motor-vehicle accidents took the lives of about 38,000 persons each year during 1959-1961—a rate of 21.2 per 100,000 persons for the three-year period—and over 48,000 in 1965. The death rate is particularly high for the age group 15-24, especially for white males (62.8 per 100,000), among whom motor vehicles are the leading cause of death and account for about one-half of all deaths. (See Appendix Table 16.)

The National Health Survey shows that over 3,000,000 persons are injured each year in moving motor-vehicle accidents. Such accidents cause about 87,000,000 days of restricted activity annually, as well as 17,000,000 workdays lost and 26,000,000 days of bed-disability. About one-fourth of the total injured are hospitalized. The prevalence of impairments from this cause is estimated at 1,500,000. Although moving motor vehicles are responsible for only about 6 percent of all estimated injuries, they account for over 20 percent of bed-days and workdays lost. The seriousness of such accidents is indicated by the fact that their victims comprise about one-third of all those hospitalized for injuries and two-fifths of those who die from injuries.

About 20 percent of the deaths and 15 percent of the injuries are to pedestrians. Because the circumstances of these accidents are very different from those causing injuries to occupants of cars, each will be considered separately.

Motor-vehicle pedestrian accidents. About 7,200 pedestrians were killed annually by motor vehicles in traffic during 1959-1961—a rate of about 4.0 per 100,000 persons (see Appendix Table 19). National Health Survey estimates show that about 14 percent of injuries from moving motor-vehicle accidents occur to persons outside the vehicle. The death rate for motor-vehicle accidents to pedestrians, as might be expected, is lowest for infants (see Appendix Table 19). It increases for each year of age, reaching a rate of about 6.0 per 100,000 for children aged 4; then it decreases with age and is lowest for the age group 15-34. After 34 it increases progressively with age again and is highest for those 85 and over. Thus, except for infants who have not learned to walk, motor-vehicle accidents to pedestrians are highest in the very young and the very old. In this respect they resemble the patterns of fires and explosions, falls and poison (Charts 4.1, 4.2, and 3.5).

The injury rate for this type of accident is highest for children under 15, but the rates are not progressively higher for elderly people—perhaps partly because an older person is very likely to be killed when struck by a motor vehicle.

The death rate for this accident type is higher for males than for females at all ages and higher for nonwhites than for whites. The age pattern is somewhat the same for all four color-sex groups (see Appendix Table 19).

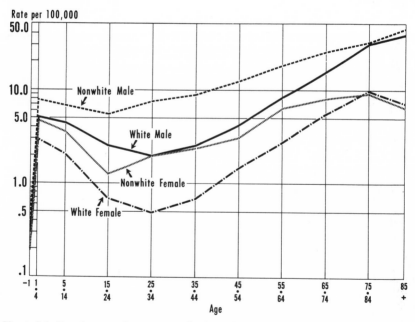

Chart 4.1. Death rates for motor-vehicle traffic accidents to pedestrians by age, color, and sex: United States, 1959-1961.

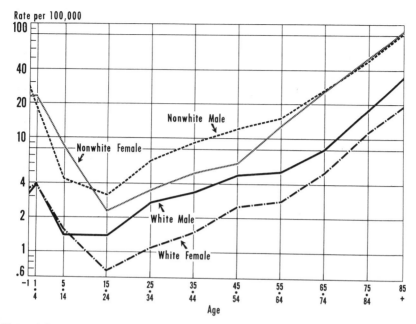

Chart 4.2. Death rates for fires and explosions by age, color, and sex: United States, 1959-1961.

Within the nonwhite group, Indians have the highest death rate from motor-vehicle accidents to pedestrians; it is almost three times that of Negroes. Chinese and Japanese have the lowest rates (see Appendix Table 13).

Among whites, the death rate to pedestrians is much higher for the foreign-born than for the native-born. This applies to all age groups, but particularly to those under 5 and over 65. (See Appendix Table 12.) White persons living in metropolitan counties that have a central city experience higher pedestrian death rates than those living in other areas (see Appendix Table 11). This may reflect the fact that the white foreign-born, with their higher death rates, are often concentrated in cities where more than half of the deaths from motor vehicles are to pedestrians. The higher rate for city-dwellers applies to white males and females. But for nonwhite males and females, the nonmetropolitan counties have the highest rates. (See Appendix Table 11.)

Among white persons, the age-adjusted death rate for pedestrians is highest geographically in the Pacific and East South Central divisions; among individual states, Arizona, New Mexico, and Nevada have the highest rates. Lowest rates are in the West North Central, New England, and East North Central areas. The highest age-adjusted death rates for nonwhites are in the Mountain, West North Central, and South Atlantic states (see Appendix Table 20), reflecting the high death rate among Indians and Negroes (Appendix Table 13). South Dakota, Utah, Wyoming, New Mexico, Idaho, and Arizona have particularly high rates (Appendix Table 20).

As in the case of many types of accidental deaths, the death rate for motor-vehicle pedestrian accidents is lowest for married persons and highest among the divorced and among widows and widowers. This is true in all age groups and among both whites and nonwhites, but it is particularly applicable to the older age groups (see Appendix Table 14).

As one might guess, deaths to pedestrians in the United States, especially to older persons, are highest during winter months. For children under 5 the peak months are those in the summer; this is also true in general for children in the 5-14 age group and it applies to both sexes and to whites and nonwhites. (See Appendix Table 15.)

Deaths from motor-vehicle accidents to pedestrians are highest by far during the hours of darkness;[2] degree of visibility is probably a major factor. Presumably, the reduction in visibility that darkness causes is more of a problem with older people than with children—especially since children go to bed earlier—and it probably accounts for the higher death rate in the winter. Dusk is a particularly dangerous time, especially for pedestrians wearing dark clothing.

The trend of pedestrian motor-vehicle deaths in the United States has been quite steadily downward since the end of World War II, with a slight increase in recent years (since 1962). Whether this increase is a temporary, cyclical affair or part of a continuing increase is not yet known; it may be related, however, to the general increase in all motor-vehicle deaths. The earlier reduction appears to have been greater in older than in younger persons; as more and more older persons drive motor vehicles, therefore, the rate could decrease still further. The smallest reduction in pedestrian deaths is among preschool children.

The literature available on pedestrian deaths and injuries contains few epidemiologic studies, but one outstanding study has been conducted by William Haddon and others on adult pedestrians fatally injured by motor vehicles in Manhattan. These pedestrians, they observed, were older than pedestrians in general, more likely to be foreign-born, less likely to be married, and of a lower socioeconomic status than those in the study control group. Most of them lived in Manhattan and were killed within a relatively short distance of their residences. Those killed had significantly higher percentages of alcohol in their blood than the control group had. It is believed that a large proportion of those with high alcohol concentrations in their blood were chronic alcoholics, but controlled observations were not possible.[3] (A discussion of pedestrian accidents from the viewpoint of host factors can be found above in "Accidents to the Aged," Chapter 3.)

Motor-vehicle nonpedestrian accidents. Most deaths and injuries from moving motor-vehicle accidents are incurred by the occupants of the cars. This was true for about 31,000 deaths annually during the period 1959-1961. The death rate for this period was 16.7 per 100,000 persons (see Appendix Table 10). There are also about 3,000,000 persons injured in such accidents each year.

Within the category of moving motor-vehicle accidents to occupants of a car, there are differences in patterns of persons killed in accidents involving running off a road, those that involve two or more vehicles, and so on. These differences will be discussed within the limits of the data available, which, unfortunately, do not distinguish between drivers and passengers of an auto.

Collisions between two or more vehicles yield the death rate 7.1 per every 100,000 persons; accidents involving running off the road, 4.5; and collisions with trains, 0.7. (See Appendix Table 17.) As will be discussed later, great variations exist in sex-age distribution for the different types of accidents. Although running off a roadway accounts for a significant portion of deaths from moving motor-vehicle accidents, almost all injuries are caused by collisions. (Some, of course, are caused by running off a roadway or striking an object on the road, or by sudden stops.)

The death rate for occupants of moving motor vehicles is higher for males than for females and, in general, for whites than for nonwhites (see Appendix Table 24 and Chart 4.3). Chart 3.4 illustrates the difference in the age distribution of white males killed in collisions and those killed in accidents involving running off the roadway. It will be noted that both kinds of deaths peak in the age group 15-24, but those involving running off the roadway decline continuously and those involving collisions decline but then increase to a peak among males aged 75. Presumably, the slowing reflexes and other character-

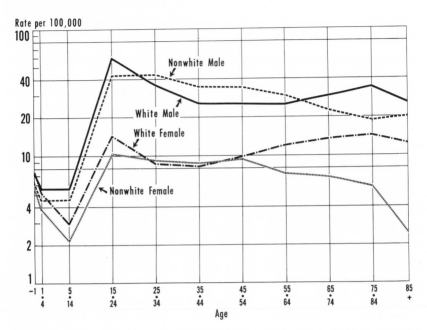

Chart 4.3. Death rates for motor-vehicle accidents other than pedestrian traffic accidents by age, color, and sex: United States, 1959-1961.

istics of age contribute to the involvement of elderly males in collisions on today's highways.

Surprising, perhaps, is the high death rate among children under 5, and especially that for infants. In children, too, the death rate for males is higher than that for females except among infants (a phenomenon already observed for other types of accidents). The lowest death rate for motor-vehicle accidents is for children aged 5-14 (see Appendix Table 24); this group has rather high rates for motor-vehicle pedestrian accidents, but presumably children of these ages do not ride with their parents as frequently as their younger brothers and sisters do and so are not exposed to the same risks. For males and females, whites and nonwhites, the highest rates are in the age group 15-24, although for nonwhite males the rate is almost equal in the group aged 25-34. Further, the rate is higher in the whites aged 15-24 than in nonwhites of the same group. Access to motor vehicles at an earlier age than among nonwhites, and the customs and mores of our society, probably account for this carnage among whites aged 15-24. (See Appendix Table 24.)

The injury rate for this type of accident is higher for males than for females (19 and 14, respectively, per 1,000 persons), although the differential is not as great as that for deaths. Again we see that the age group 15-24—males and females, both—has the highest injury rate for moving vehicles (National Health Survey). Among males aged 15-24, who have been involved in such accidents, more drivers have been injured than passengers; but among females the number of passengers is much higher than that of drivers. The injury rate to passengers aged 15-24 is higher than in other age groups and is even higher than the injury rate for drivers, which does not vary much with age.

It is interesting to observe the difference between the patterns of deaths and injuries by age and sex for nonpedestrian motor-vehicle accidents. Both peak in the age group 15-24, but not nearly as much for injuries as for deaths. Chart 4.4 shows the ratio of injuries to deaths for males and females by age. It is noteworthy that for very young children the ratio of injuries to deaths is rather low, indicating a high case fatality rate. For school children the high ratio of injuries to deaths indicates that injuries are much less likely to be fatal in that group; but in the age group 15-24, the ratio of injuries to deaths (for males) is extremely low again, indicating the very high case fatality rate. This latter low ratio resembles somewhat the ratio pattern for firearms (Chart 4.5) and may indicate some similarity between the causation of motor-vehicle deaths on the highways and that of firearm accidents among males of this age group. The ratio for females in the same age group does not show as drastic a decrease as for males. For both males and females, the ratio of injuries to deaths declines in older groups, again indicating the increased likelihood among older persons of death from injury. As is true for other types of injuries, the ratio of injuries to deaths is higher for females than males at all ages except in the preschool child.

Among nonwhites, Indians have the highest death rate for this type of accident and Negroes the second highest. Japanese and Chinese have the lowest rates—as they do for almost every type of accident (see Appendix Table 13).

The native-born white has a higher death rate for nonpedestrian motor-vehicle accidents than does the foreign-born white. Among children under five, however, the reverse is true—as it is for deaths to pedestrians, from falls and other causes. It appears that the native-born excess rises among older groups (see Appendix Table 12).

In the section "Race, Color, Place of Birth" (Chapter 3), motor-

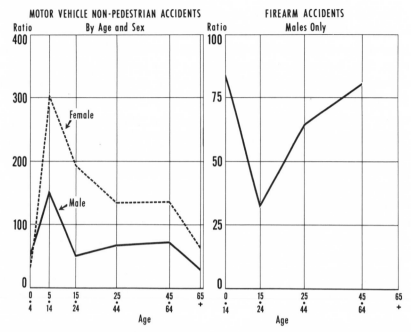

Chart 4.4. Ratio of injuries to deaths for motor-vehicle nonpedestrian accidents by age and sex: United States, 1959-1961. Sources: deaths—Division of Vital Statistics, National Center for Health Statistics, 1959-1961; injuries—Division of Health Interview Statistics, National Center for Health Statistics, July 1959-June 1961.

Chart 4.5. Ratio of injuries to deaths for firearm accidents—males only; United States, 1959-1961. Sources: deaths—Division of Vital Statistics, National Center for Health Statistics, 1959-1961; injuries—Division of Health Interview Statistics, July 1959-June 1961.

vehicle accident death rates for foreign-born whites were presented by country of origin; it was pointed out that among residents of the United States, persons born in Mexico have the highest rate for foreign groups and those born in Italy the lowest.

Married persons of all sex-race groups and all ages, have the lowest death rate as occupants of motor vehicles (see Appendix Table 14), as is true of deaths from other types of accidents and other causes. There are two exceptions: older persons, and males under 20. In the age group under 20, the rate for married males is higher than that for single males; in females it is about the same for both (see Appendix

Table 25). As mentioned earlier, it is possible that married males under 20 are atypical and are thus exposed to a higher accident death rate—just as it is possible that the high death rate for widows and widowers, especially in the younger age groups, is due to an artifact (when both parties die in the same automobile accident the second party to die may be classified as a widow or widower on the death certificate). In the older age groups, especially female, the rate for those married is higher than that for those single: elderly married women probably tend to drive with their husbands, whereas their single counterparts might not be expected to drive as often.

Death rates to occupants of an automobile appear to be highest, geographically, in the Mountain division and lowest in the New England and Middle Atlantic states. Nevada has the highest rate in the country and Rhode Island the lowest (see Appendix Table 23). Injury data available from the National Health Survey for four large regions of the United States show that the West has the highest rate (male and female) by far; this is true for all age groups, although data are not available for age by sex. An interesting phenomenon—for which there is no obvious explanation—is the higher injury rate for females than for males in the West.

Unlike death rates for pedestrians, the rate for occupants of a car is higher in nonmetropolitan counties for whites and nonwhites, males and females. It is higher for whites in counties having a central city than in counties without a central city, but for nonwhites the pattern is reversed. (See Appendix Table 11.)

According to the National Health Survey, rural nonfarm residents, both male and female, have the highest nonpedestrian motor-vehicle injury rates; rural farm and urban rates are about the same.

There is little seasonal variation in death rates for occupants of a motor vehicle when all ages are considered. It would appear that the large amount of traveling done in the summer is balanced by poor driving conditions in the winter. But among children there does seem to be an excess of deaths in the summer months; with increasing age, the higher rates move toward the months of November and December. Although driving conditions in January are somewhat more unfavorable than in December, January's rates are extremely low; the irregular circumstances of the December holiday season may be involved.

After reaching a peak in the late 1930's and early 1940's, the death rate for moving motor vehicles has remained relatively steady. From 1962 through 1965 an annual increase in deaths to occupants of motor vehicles was noted, however, both in rate and in numbers, and a new high in numbers was reached in 1965. Preliminary figures for 1966 have shown a continuing increase. Injury rates and, interestingly enough, deaths from the inhalation of automobile exhaust gas, have shown similar increases in recent years.

Contributory factors. In no accident field has so much research been carried out on causative factors as in the epidemiology of motor-vehicle accidents. For the sake of organization, these accidents will be discussed very briefly under the categories of host, agent, and environment. Much overlapping of data must be assumed, especially in considering cultural and social factors.

One approach to such epidemiologic investigation involves the use of teams of experts in different fields like medicine, engineering, and social science. Typical of this approach is the study carried out by J. S. Baker at Northwestern University.[4] Some approaches involve a kind of control group, as in Haddon's investigations in New York;[5] and others involve the determination of characteristics of drivers by categorizing groups and observing and comparing their driving experiences (studies by John Conger[6] and Frederick McGuire,[7] for example).

Variables chosen to measure the "accident" range from death to traffic violations and include combinations of separate variables. It is sometimes assumed that if one could learn both the characteristics of drivers who violate laws or become involved in property damage accidents (or even accidents involving only minor injuries) and the circumstances under which such violations and accidents occur, one would have identified the etiology of fatal accidents. But this may be a dangerous assumption.

To illustrate the differences in distribution of injuries and deaths to occupants of automobiles, a ratio of injuries to deaths (the inverse of the case fatality rate) has been calculated for different circumstances and presented in Charts 4.4 and 4.6. As mentioned earlier, Chart 4.4 shows the low ratio for males aged 15-24 and illustrates the severity of injuries incurred by this group. For both sexes the ratios are low among older groups. Chart 4.6 gives ratios computed by time of day; the seriousness of injuries incurred late at night and very early in the morning is evident. Differences have also been observed by geography, urbanization, weather and road conditions, kinds of roads, and other variables. All of the differences should be considered by researchers and others studying variables in motor-vehicle accidents.

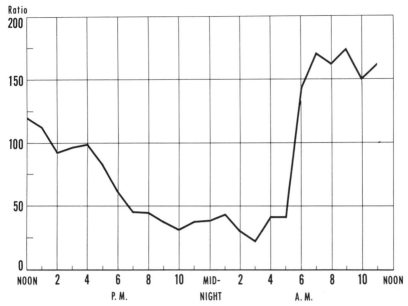

Chart 4.6. Ratio of injuries to deaths for motor-vehicle accidents by time of day (three-hour moving average). Source: Facts: 1961 (Hartford: Connecticut Department of Motor Vehicles).

Much research has been concerned with the attempt to identify the "accident prone" or "susceptible" drivers, or those more likely to become involved in accidents than the average driver. The literature is summarized well by McFarland, Moore, and Warren,[8] and by Leon Goldstein.[9] Merriam and Quint, after reviewing the literature on contributory factors involved in motor-vehicle accidents, list a number of characteristic adjectives that appear to be associable with high and low accident groups.[10]

The many variables involved are apparent from even a cursory review of the literature; but ways of life, inability to adjust to demands of life or culture, and influence of peers and cultural patterns emerge as outstanding factors, as opposed to what are termed "single attributes," no matter how they are measured. Among the factors considered and discussed in "Host Factors" (Chapter 3) are sensory abilities (especially vision); psychomotor capacity; cognition; personal, emotional, and attitudinal factors; fatigue; drugs, medications, and other toxic substances. The role of alcohol is referred to with increasing frequency, and alcoholism or problem-drinking, as well as social drinking, is emphasized. Psychiatric conditions are also being discussed, as an addition to temporary emotional upsets.

There is increasing emphasis on vehicle design and the role of defects that appear both in design and through mechanical failure. Brakes, windshield wipers, headlights and back-up lights, visibility factors, types and location of controls, as well as features designed to modify effects of impact, are being studied and improved.

The Cornell Crash Injury Project is concerned with injuries to occupants of cars through the impact of the human body with objects inside and outside the car; the study of structure and design of cars and restraining devices is, therefore, involved. Data are volunteered by police departments, medical societies, departments of public health, motor-vehicle departments, hospital associations, and other organizations; the source of the data is rural areas. The Project's findings provide a sounder knowledge of injury causation, as well as information regarding methods of eliminating the causes or lessening their gravity. The knowledge gained has been helpful in developing such features as seat belts, improved door locks, energy-absorbing steering wheels, and padded instrument panels.[11]

The design of highways for both high-speed and local travel, with attention to visibility and illumination, traffic signs and signals, anti-skid surfaces, and protection against monotony, is important for safety as well as for the facilitation of traffic flow.

The restriction of driving privileges—through licensing procedures, for example—whether for driving experience (violations or accidents) or characteristics of the driver (problems of age, medical conditions, and so on) is being given increasing attention by motor-vehicle administrators. Because of this, of course, questions of administration as well as of rights and legal implications are raised.

The interaction of host, agent and environment should again be emphasized, as should the fact that characteristics of the host considered unsafe under some circumstances (at night, or while driving at high speed) may not be unsafe under others.

Motorcycle accidents
Deaths from motorcycle accidents are to drivers and passengers (pillion and sidecar, both) of motorcycles, motorized cycles, and motorized scooters. In the United States in 1960 there were about 730 deaths from motorcycle accidents—a rate of 0.4 per 100,000 persons.

Most of these deaths involved collisions in traffic with other motor vehicles (62 percent). The only other category with a large number of deaths was that of noncollision traffic accidents (32 percent), which includes such accidents as overturning or running off the roadway. The remainder were in the categories nontraffic accidents and "traffic accidents—collision with nonmotor vehicle or object."

Deaths from motorcycle accidents occur to persons of all ages, but the highest rates are in the 15-29 group. About 93 percent occur to males. Such deaths are most frequent in the summer months.

Motorcycle accidents were first categorized separately in the International Code in 1949. The death rate that year was 0.7 per 100,000; it decreased to 0.4 in 1954, remaining about the same until 1963, when it rose to 0.5 and then to 0.6 in 1964. The number of deaths in 1949 was 1,103, decreasing to 600-750 annually during the period 1953-1961; thereafter it increased to the 1965 estimate of 1,580 deaths.

Information from various sources shows that the head and lower limbs are frequently injured (and fractured) in motorcycle accidents. Head injuries are usually serious, often fatal. The advisability of wearing a safety helmet while riding a motorcycle or motor scooter is emphasized increasingly.

Many investigations have shown that some persons begin riding without any training; also, many riders use rented or borrowed cycles.

In 1960 there were almost 575,000 registered motorcycles, but by the end of 1965 registrations had risen to more than 1,380,000.

Pedal-cycle accidents

A pedal cycle is a road-transport vehicle operated solely by pedals, other than a child's tricycle.[12] Riders and passengers of pedal cycles—primarily bicycles—can become involved in five classifications of death statistics. In two of these there are very few deaths (motor-vehicle nontraffic accidents to pedal cyclists and accidents to occupants of motor vehicles in collision with pedestrians or pedal cycles), and they are not included in the following analysis.

The majority of pedal-cycle deaths are from motor-vehicle traffic accidents to pedal cyclists (450 deaths in 1960 alone), included in the category motor-vehicle accidents. Other road-vehicle accidents include accidents to pedestrians by pedal cycles, and accidents to pedal-cycle riders not involving collisions with motor vehicles. In these groups there were 67 deaths in 1960, of which 16 were to pedestrians. The total number of pedal-cycle deaths has increased from around 400 (0.2 per 100,000 persons) in the early 1950's to over 600 in 1963 (0.3).

According to estimates from the Division of Accident Prevention of the Public Health Service, approximately a million persons are injured each year in bicycle accidents. Most injuries are to youngsters and most to males. The problem of injuries from bicycle collisions with motor vehicles is obvious. Not so apparent, however, is the large number of injuries from other types of accidents to bicyclers. In a study of the circumstances surrounding nonmotor-vehicle accidents to children under 15, it was found that the practice of riding double, defective or inadequate equipment, inexperience, use of a bicycle too large for its rider, loss of balance, and inattention were factors that, alone or in combination, had produced the accidents. The most frequent single contributing factor was that of gravelly, slippery, or uneven surfaces. Also, of course, bicyclers can be injured in collisions with other bicycles.[13]

The National Safety Council has studied fatal bicycle accidents involving motor vehicles for the year 1957. In almost two-thirds of the accidents a violation was committed by the pedal cyclist; in approximately one-third of the violations the cyclist did not have the right of way. In most of the accidents the motor vehicle was moving straight ahead, not turning: about 70 percent of the accidents occurred during the daylight hours.[14]

Aircraft accidents

Death statistics for aircraft accidents include accidental deaths to persons aboard military and civil aircraft, to persons boarding and alighting, and to those not actually in aircraft but killed as a result of aircraft accidents. There are about 1,400 deaths from aircraft accidents each year in the United States: a rate of 0.8 per 100,000 persons (see Appendix Table 10). About 300 are to persons in military aircraft (0.2), about 300 in commercial aircraft (0.2), and about 800 in "general aviation" (0.5), which includes such categories as pleasure, business, and instruction. Fatalities are about equally divided between pilots and passengers.

The death rate is very low for age groups under 15 (0.1 per 100,000) but increases to a peak in the age group 25-34 (2.1); thereafter it decreases, until for ages 75 and over the rate is 0.1. The rate for white males, 1.6, is by far the highest of the four color-sex groups (see Appendix Table 10).

From 1930 to 1941 the death rate was quite low, ranging between 0.3 and 0.6. During the war years 1942-1945 the rate was much higher—between 2.2 and 5.3—and in 1946 it was 1.3. There has been, since then, a gradual reduction to 0.8 in 1964. Since 1960 a reduction has occurred in deaths in scheduled air service and an increase in deaths in general aviation.

The small number of fatal accidents and the relatively larger number of passenger fatalities in some accidents result in fatality rates that are subject to marked fluctuation from year to year. The rates that follow, therefore, are averages of several years: in the United States, the passenger death rate per 1,000 passenger hours for scheduled airlines was 0.0011 for 1952-1964; for supplemental airlines it was 0.004 for 1956-1963; for general aviation it was 0.008 for 1956-1962. For the same periods, respectively, the "first pilot" death rate per 1,000 airplane hours was 0.0013 for scheduled airlines, 0.005 for supplemental, and 0.007 for general.[15]

The Federal Aviation Agency studied one-third of the fatal accidents in general aviation for 1963. Of the pilots involved, 35 percent were "positive" in investigations for blood and/or tissue alcohol. The study revealed a much higher prevalence of proven alcohol intake than previously known.[16]

The Parachute Club of America reports that during 1961-1965 there were 125 deaths to persons participating in sport parachuting or skydiving. The Club estimates that there are 25,000-30,000 active participants.[17]

Drowning

Deaths by drowning fall into two principal categories: accidental drowning and submersion and water-transport deaths. The former includes all drownings except those in water-transport accidents. About 90 percent of the latter result either from the submersion of an occupant of a small boat (passenger capacity of less than ten) or from other water-transport injuries by submersion. Some drownings occur in nonwater-transport accidents, but they are few in number: about 5 percent of deaths from aircraft accidents, for instance, are drownings. A special tabulation prepared by the Illinois Department of Public Health for the period 1957-1961 shows that about 2 percent of two types of motor-vehicle accidents result in drowning: collisions with fixed objects and accidents involving running off the roadway.

About 7 percent of all accidental deaths are drownings of the types included in the two principal categories. These rank fourth as a cause of accidental death in the United States, having rates of 2.9 per

100,000 persons for drowning and submersion and about 0.8 for water-transport accidents (see Appendix Table 10). Each year about 6,500 persons drown—about 1,300 in water-transport accidents and 5,200 from nontransport accidents.

Because the data available for nontransport drownings are more specific than for water-transport deaths, these types of accidents will be discussed separately; but many reports other than from death certificates combine the two into a single category.

Nontransport drownings. The infant death rate in this category is about 1.4 per 100,000; the rate at age 1, however, is 6.1—higher than for any other age group. The rate gradually lowers through age 4, but it increases to 4.7 in the 15-24 group. Between this age and the group 85 and over (where it is slightly higher) the rate is about 2.0 (see Appendix Table 33). Family swimming pools are an increasing problem with regard to preschool children.

Nonwhite persons have a higher drowning rate than do white persons, and males a much higher rate than females. Except for infants, however, the drowning rate is higher in white preschool children than in nonwhite (see Appendix Table 33). Nonwhite males have the highest rate—9.8 per 100,000—followed by white males with a rate of 4.3, nonwhite females at 1.1 and white females at 0.9; the same pattern exists when the rates are adjusted according to age (see Appendix Table 35). There are over 5 male deaths from drowning for each female death, but there is considerable variation in this ratio by age: among infants the ratio is about 1 to 1, increasing to about 12 to 1 in the age group 15-24; it then declines to about 3 to 1 in the age group 85 and over.

Nonwhites have a drowning rate of 5.3 per 100,000, but there are substantial differences by race. Chinese and Japanese have the lowest rates (2.1 and 3.7 respectively); Negroes have a rate of 5.2; and Indians have the highest rate, 12.3. (See Appendix Table 13.)

The death rate for foreign-born whites is higher than for native-born whites, particularly in males. This difference is most apparent in the younger and older age groups, where the rates for foreign-born males are two to three times those of the native-born. For example, the age-adjusted rates for male children under 15 are 10.7 per 100,000 for the foreign-born and 4.8 for the native-born; age-adjusted rates for males 65 and over are 6.0 for the foreign-born and 3.7 for the native-born.

The "place" coded on death certificates for nontransport accidents is not particularly appropriate for recording drownings at beaches, lakes, rivers, seashores, and other places not designated as sites of recreation and sports. All of these fall into the category "other specified places," under which 70 percent of the drownings are listed (see Appendix Table 38). (The exception is the preschool child: most drownings in this age group occur at home or on farms.) About 15 percent of drownings in school-age children occur in places for recreation and sport; otherwise, the bulk of drownings occur in unorganized and unsupervised areas. About one-fourth of all white female drownings occur on "home premises"; but this is an infrequent site for drownings of white males who are of school age or older.

Alaska has the highest drowning rate (11.9 per 100,000) and Rhode Island the lowest (1.7). In general, the highest rates are in the South Atlantic and Mountain states and the lowest in the Middle Atlantic, North Central, and New England states. There are low rates in the band of states starting with Massachusetts, Connecticut, Rhode Island, and New Jersey and extending westward through Nebraska and Kansas. High and moderately high rates are found in the Southeastern Atlantic states (below Maryland) and the Gulf Coast states. (See Appendix Table 34.)

Residents of nonmetropolitan counties have higher death rates for drowning than do those of metropolitan counties. Among infants and the aged, however, the highest rates are in metropolitan areas with a central city (see Appendix Table 11).

Drownings, as would be expected, are highest in the summer months; the peak occurs in July (see Appendix Table 15). The seasonal pattern is more pronounced in younger than in older persons, indicating the predominant role played by recreation in drownings among young persons.

As was true for deaths from all accidents, married persons of both sexes, white and nonwhite, have the lowest rate for drowning. Divorced males and widowers have the highest age-adjusted rates (11.7 per 100,000); married males have the lowest (3.0); and single males have a rate of 8.8. In women, widows have the highest rate (2.6), followed by divorced females (1.6); single females have a rate of 0.8 and those married 0.4. For males 65 and over, the age-adjusted death rate is highest for those divorced and next highest for those single, followed by widowers and those who are married.

Water-transport drownings. Most water-transport deaths involve the drowning of occupants of small boats. Nearly all these deaths are to males: 1.6 per 100,000 persons, compared with 0.1 for females (see Appendix Table 10). Nonwhite males have higher rates than white males in all age groups. The rate for very young males is low, but it rises in the age group 5-14. For white males, the rate is highest in the 15-24 group (2.5 per 100,000), decreasing slightly in each age group thereafter; the rate for nonwhite males increases to a high of 3.6 for the 45-54 age group and decreases thereafter.

General drownings. Bramwell Gabrielson has reported that in 1955 about 33 percent of drownings in the United States occurred in lakes and nearly 30 percent in rivers; large numbers of drownings also occurred in streams, creeks, ponds, dammed waters, oceans, bays, and sounds.[18] Localities vary among states, depending upon their topographical characteristics. Seemingly harmless locations may contain drowning potentials, particularly when small children are involved.

In recent years there has been a change in the prominence of some places over others as locations of drownings. Warren Morse has estimated, for instance, that 62 drownings occurred in home swimming pools in the United States in 1958.[19] In 1963, California alone reported 100 such deaths[20] and Florida recorded 23.[21] An important factor in the California experience was the age of the victims: over half were preschool children, and one-fourth were infants.

An insurance company study of drownings in children aged 1-4 reports that preoccupied adults too often forget that active children must be watched constantly. In many of the cases studied, drowning occurred while parents or other adults supervised a child's play from indoors; by the time the child's disappearance was noticed it was too late for rescue. About one-third of the victims drowned at home and almost as many a short distance from home.[22]

It is difficult to ascertain the frequency of particular types of accidents involving drowning, for few studies contain complete information on this subject. Twenty-six percent of the drownings covered in Gabrielson's study occurred while swimming, 19 percent while fishing, 16 percent while boating, and 17 percent while "wandering, walking, exploring, or playing and falling into water from dock, bridge, shore, etc." Also cited are hunting, "walking or playing on thin ice," water skiing, skin or scuba diving, and bathing.[23]

The United States Coast Guard publishes annual reports on accidents in recreational boating in this country. In the 1964 edition it was reported that of 1,772 persons "in peril in the water," 1,192 died. Almost 90 percent of the deaths were from drowning. Other victims, in the water, died from other causes or disappeared; contributing factors included lack of adequate lifesaving devices, failure to use available devices, and inability to swim. Most of the craft involved in the accidents were motorboats less than 16 feet long. Of the 1,772 persons in peril, 33 percent were rescued. The chance of being rescued improved from 28 percent for those without lifesaving devices to 57 percent for those using such devices. Sixty percent of those with devices survived, while only 20 percent of those without them survived. The swimming ability of over half of the persons in peril was unknown; but of those for whom such information was available, the chance for survival increased among good or fair swimmers.[24]

California identified 21 drownings from skin and scuba diving in 1963, and Florida 17 from skin diving in 1962. G. D. Taylor and others have canvassed all State Vital Statistics only to find information on drownings of this kind unavailable in the majority of states. However, they did uncover information on 37 skin and scuba diving deaths that had occurred during a 32-month period (January 1960-August 1962) in Florida. All but one of these deaths were due to drowning; the other involved an attack by a shark. Two-thirds of the deaths occurred in springs formed by underground rivers that surface through caves, the remainder in ocean waters. Most of the divers were with "buddies," but they were not always in close proximity. The researchers have concluded an exhausted air supply was a major factor in the causes of most of the accidents; only a few victims were wearing depth gauges or diving watches. Ocean deaths were attributed in part to a combination of ocean currents and lack of safety lines.[25]

The California Department of Public Health does not completely agree with these conclusions about causes. In a report by its Bureau of Occupational Health, the Department states: "It is generally felt that simple drowning is the most frequent cause of death in scuba diving. Although the various gases involved in the scuba diver's body system may contribute to setting the stage for drowning to occur, panic and exhaustion appear to be the major related factors."[26]

A report from Michigan shows that in 21 deaths from scuba diving 15 divers were inexperienced, 3 were diving for the first time, and 3 had been receiving instruction. Eighteen of the deaths were in water a depth of 25 feet or less. Ten divers drowned; 11 deaths were diagnosed as pulmonary barotrauma, with air embolism as the probable agent of death.[27]

Conflicting opinions in these reports on causation would seem to indicate the need for careful autopsies.

In Gabrielson's study, the two major causes of drowning are "falling out of boat or boat capsizing" (24 percent) and "child unattended, wandered or fell into water" (17 percent). Other causes include: "stepped in hole or dropped off while swimming, wading, or fishing" (6 percent); "poor swimmers—tried to swim too far for their ability" (4 percent); "nonswimmer or poor swimmer, swimming in area not patrolled" (10 percent); and "fell into water from dock, bridge, rocks, shore, etc." (10 percent).[28]

In a study of Iowa drownings, causes mentioned frequently included exhaustion or physical attack (23 percent); falling from a bank (18 percent); stepping into deep water (13 percent); sinking of a boat (10 percent); falling into a tank or well (8 percent); falling from a boat (7 percent); and falling from a pier, dock, or bridge (5 percent).[29]

The studies of boating accidents mentioned earlier indicate that the ability to swim improves one's chances of survival. Gabrielson reports that 71 percent of the drowning victims in his study were nonswimmers and only about 5 percent were good or excellent swimmers.[30]

In spite of increased facilities for and activities involving water recreation, death rates from drowning have declined steadily over the years for both nontransport and transport drownings and have shown about a 20 percent reduction in the last decade.

Poisoning by solid or liquid substances

Each year in the United States about 1,700 deaths occur from poisoning by solid or liquid substances, a rate of 1.0 per 100,000 persons (see Appendix Table 10). A large proportion of these deaths (about 450) are among preschool children; the infant rate is 1.3, and the rate for children aged 1-4 is 2.4. (See Appendix Table 37.) Children under 5 also have the highest estimated injury rate from swallowing poisonous substances. Deaths from poisoning are low in school children and young persons, but the rate begins to rise again at about age 35.

It should be noted at the outset that death from accidental poisoning does not in this discussion include the following: deaths in which continued intake has caused a condition like alcoholism or chronic poisoning from narcotics, and deaths from food poisoning of bacterial origin (by infection or intoxication)—botulism, for example. Accidental poisoning by solid and liquid substance does include poisoning by noxious foodstuffs.

Males have a higher death rate from this cause than do females, in general, and the nonwhite rate is higher than that for whites (see Appendix Table 37). Among nonwhites, the Indian rate is highest and the Chinese and Japanese lowest (see Appendix Table 13).

In about 85 percent of the poisoning deaths for which place of occurrence is specified on the death certificate, the place is the home (see Appendix Table 38). Most nonfatal poisoning also occurs in the home.

The South Atlantic area has the highest age-adjusted death rate and the West North Central the lowest. Data are not available by geographic area for nonfatal incidents.

There have not been many changes in death rates for these types of poisoning in the past two decades because increases in the numbers of deaths have been offset by the growing population. The rate was 1.1 per 100,000 persons in 1949; it decreased to 0.8 and gradually increased again to 1.1 in 1963 and 1964. There were over 1,600 of these deaths in 1949; this figure decreased to 1,400 and then gradually increased to 2,100 in 1964. Deaths among persons aged 15 and over, rather than among children under 15, account for the increases in recent years. The number of deaths for children in the 1-4 group decreased by 14 percent from 1960 to 1964.

The National Clearinghouse for Poison Control Centers in the Division of Accident Prevention of the Public Health Service receives reports from poison control centers located throughout the United States. Approximately 90 percent of the accidental ingestions reported to the Clearinghouse are for children under 5; the discussion hereafter will therefore be limited to that group. Because of rapid changes between the stages of growth and development of children in their earlier years, descriptions of differences in the patterns of poisoning in children will be given by 6-month periods. The age at which poisoning is apparently most frequent is 18-24 months. Almost one-fourth of the incidents in children under 5 occur in this 6-month period; about three-fourths are in the group aged 12-36 months.

There are differences in the types of products ingested by children in different age groups. Household cleaning and polishing agents, pesticides, petroleum-distillate products, and paints and paint solvents are ingested most frequently by one-year-olds. Two-year-olds ingest medications more often than do children in other age groups: 39 percent of all external medication and 46 percent of all internal medication ingestions involve two-year-old children. But the proportion of poisoning from internal medicine is higher in older children: as children grow older they become more discriminating in their tastes, and the pattern changes from external to internal medication. This increase continues with age from 16 percent of poisonings in children under one to 55 percent in four-year-olds. (See Chart 4.7.)

Aspirin comprises about 50 percent of the internal medicine ingested and is involved in one-fifth of all poisoning accidents. In cases where the type of aspirin is known, the "baby" type figures in about 80 percent of poisonings.[31] Investigations into surrounding circumstances have revealed that poisonous substances ingested, especially petroleum products, are often not in their original containers or their usual places of storage.

As is true of many accident categories, the type of product ingested is related to socioeconomic status, cultural patterns, geography, weather, and other factors. Medicine, for example, appears more frequently in well-to-do than in poorer homes. In general, medicines are ingested more frequently in the Northeast and Great Lakes areas; a high pro-

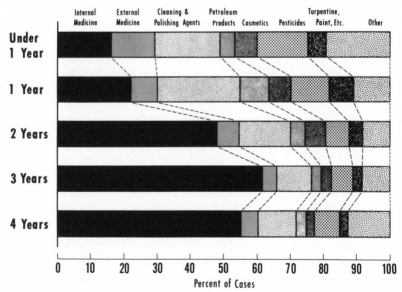

Chart 4.7. Type of product as a percentage of all accidental ingestion among children under 5 years of age: 1959-1961. Source: Individual poison reports by 243 poison control centers in 38 states.

portion of ingestions in southern states consists of petroleum distillates and pesticides. Within the home, the kitchen is the most frequent place of ingestion.

Lead, a major problem in the poisoning of small children, may be present in many products; most often it is ingested by children eating paint in old, substandard houses. Often the paint is flaking or peeling, particularly off walls, ceilings, and windowsills. An unusual appetite for inedible substances (pica) exists in some children; this may cause them to eat the peeling paint, or dirt into which flaking paint has fallen. Lead-ingestion poisoning is chronic and may be difficult to recognize; if the physician is aware of the predisposing environmental conditions in the child's neighborhood its recognition is facilitated.

The poisoning of adults involves motivation problems that are frequently complicated by overindulgence in alcohol and by dubious suicide; the problem is not amenable to discussion in this volume.

Poisoning by gases or vapors

Approximately 1,200 persons die each year from poisoning by gases or vapors (mostly carbon monoxide)—a rate of 0.7 per 100,000 persons (see Appendix Table 10). No estimate for injuries exists. The age group 75 and over has the highest death rate for males and females, whites and nonwhites, with the nonwhite rate slightly higher than the white at all ages. The male rate is also higher than the female rate at all ages (see Appendix Table 37). The Indian rate is higher than rates of other nonwhite groups, and Chinese and Japanese rates are lowest (see Appendix Table 13).

About 70 percent of these deaths (with specified locations) occur in the home. The next most frequent places of occurrence are the street and highway (7 percent) and industrial places and premises (7 percent). (See Appendix Table 38.) The Mountain division has the highest age-adjusted death rate, the South Atlantic and Pacific areas the lowest. Seventy percent of these deaths occur during the months of November-March (see Appendix Table 15).

The death rate for gases and vapors decreased from 1.1 per 100,000 persons in 1949 to 0.7 in 1964, because of a decrease in the rate for utility (illuminating) gas from 0.6 to 0.1. The rate from motor-vehicle exhaust gas was 0.2 from 1949 to 1960, but in recent years there has been an increase to 0.3 (in 1964); deaths attributed to this cause increased from 385 in 1959 to 640 in 1964. There has been little change in the death rate from other sources of carbon monoxide gas.

Falls

About 19,000 persons die each year from falls—the second leading cause of accidental death, with a rate of 10.5 per 100,000 persons (see Appendix Table 27). Additional deaths like those involving falls in front of cars on the highway or falls from water and land transport into water (resulting in drowning), as well as others, are not assigned by the International Classification to the category of "falls." Almost three-quarters of all deaths from falls are to persons 65 and older; as many as nearly three-fifths are to those 75 and over.

Falls cause more injuries than any other type of accident. In contrast to deaths from falls, however, injuries incurred by falls are mostly the problem of youth. The National Health Survey reports that of the approximately 12,000,000 persons injured each year by falls (68 per 1000) over 40 percent are under 15 years old. Injury rates are also high among the elderly.

Accidents involving falls cause 173,000,000 days of restricted activity annually, of which there are 43,000,000 bed-disability days and 24,000,000 work-loss days. Of the 12,000,000 injured, about 10,000,000 persons receive medical attention and 3,000,000 are bed-disabled—about one-third of all persons bed-disabled because of injuries.

Approximately one-fourth of the injuries from falls are sprains or strains, 23 percent are lacerations and abrasions, and 23 percent are contusions. Head injuries including skull fractures amount to about 8 percent of the injuries, fractures of the femur about 1 percent and other fractures 13 percent. A special tabulation prepared by the Illinois Department of Public Health for the period 1957-1961 shows that fractures were the resulting injury in 77 percent of the deaths from falls. Twenty percent were from fractures of the skull and face and 47 percent from fractures of the lower limbs; 14 percent were head injuries other than skull fractures and 5 percent were injuries of internal organs.

Division of Accident Prevention studies show that falls are the leading cause of accidental injury to children. As a percentage of all injuries sustained, they steadily decrease as the child gets older: they comprise about 50 percent of all injuries to infants; 45 percent in the 1-4 group; 35 percent in children 5-9; 25 percent for ages 10-14; and 15 percent in the group 15-19.

Children under five, especially those under one, have a much higher death rate for falls than do older children (see Appendix Table 27).

Possibly young children are more predisposed to severe injury-pro-
ducing incidents and less able to withstand trauma than older children. Injuries from falls are most likely to be fatal at both extremes
of life. Chart 4.8 shows the ratio of injuries to deaths by sex and age.
In the age group under five the ratio is about 5,000 to 1, but in the
age group 15-24 it is about 24,000 to 1 for females and 12,000 to 1
for males. In the older groups it is extremely low for both sexes. At
all ages except among the very old, the ratio is lower (case fatality
rate higher) for males than for females.

The young child is exposed to hazards with which he has had no
prior experience. Epidemiologic studies by the Division of Accident
Prevention confirm what parents already know—that during the crawl-
ing stage the child under two frequently climbs upon and then falls
from such objects as chairs, sofas, and other furniture. While learning
to walk, tripping hazards are very significant: in the age group under
five the slightest surface deviation, like a turned-up rug, may cause a
fall. Nearly one-fifth of the falls resulting in injury of children under
four involve stairs or steps, another major hazard for the very young.

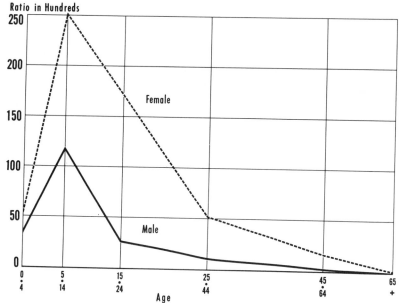

Chart 4.8. Ratio of injuries to deaths for all fall accidents by age and sex: United
States, 1959-1961. Sources: deaths—Division of Vital Statistics, National Center
for Health Statistics, 1959-1961; injuries—Division of Health Interview Statistics,
National Center for Health Statistics, July 1959-June 1961.

In the 5-9 age group the pattern of falls is altered because the child is exposed to hazards beyond the walls of the home. At this age he shows an even greater proclivity for climbing onto higher and higher objects; injuries from falls on stairs or steps become less of a problem. There is a marked decrease in accidental falls in the group 10-14. Not only are death and injury rates lowest for this age group, but the case fatality rate is also lowest.

Increased involvement in sports on the part of the 15-24 age group is apparent by the activities associable with their falls. Division of Accident Prevention investigations show that one-third of the hospitalized, treated falls in this group result from participation in some form of athletic activity. Slipping, as might be expected, seems to be a major source of injuries from falls.

Women 15 to 44 years of age are generally involved in accidental falls from one level to another (down stairs for example); men tend to fall off ladders and from other high places.

Injury and death rates display rapid increases with age for persons 65 and over. This group as a whole has an injury rate of 90 per 1,000 persons (National Health Survey); its death rates are 29.5 per 100,000 for ages 65-74, 125.4 for 75-84, and 510.8 for 85 and over. (See Appendix Table 27 and Charts 4.9 and 3.5.)

In a Division of Accident Prevention study carried out in a northeastern community on accidental injuries to elderly persons, about 85 percent of the injuries were caused by falls, and fractured hips were common especially in females. Causes of falls, especially those occurring indoors, are particularly baffling among the elderly. The victims frequently attribute them to uneven floors, protruding furniture, tripping over rugs, and sometimes dizziness and weakness; often, however, the victim is unable to explain the cause.

In another study carried out by the Division a large number of the fractured hip incidents, especially in elderly females, could not be related to obvious causal factors.[32] It was hypothesized that many of these fractures were associated with osteoporosis; this hypothesis is now being tested in a cooperative study with Ford Hospital in Detroit.[33]

Trevor Howell recognizes several other physiological conditions that can precipitate falls. He cites the shuffling tendency in old men which often results in tripping falls, and attributes this condition to inoperable growths that cause muscle weakness and inability to lift the feet.[34]

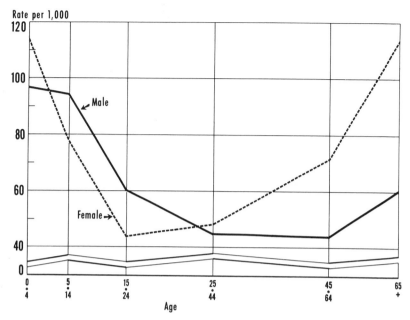

Chart 4.9. Injury rates for fall accidents by age and sex: United States 1959-1961. Source: Division of Health Interview Statistics, National Center for Health Statistics, July 1959-June 1961.

Various studies of falls in elderly persons, especially some that have been conducted in England, suggest that changes in the central nervous system are in many cases responsible for loss of balance and falls. Boucher states that "in old people, balance and the maintenance of posture is one of the first functions to disappear, and it disappears at an earlier age and more completely in women than in men."[35]

Contrary to the pattern of all accidental deaths in general, the rate for falls is greater for white persons than for nonwhites (see Appendix Table 27). Indians have the highest death rate for nonwhites, followed by Negroes, Chinese, and Japanese (Appendix Table 13). When these rates are examined by age, however, it is noted that nonwhites of both sexes have higher rates during early childhood and during the working years of life, and somewhat lower rates after age 65, than do whites. (See Appendix Table 27 and Chart 3.5.) This dramatic change in the color-sex pattern is unique in the accident picture and suggests that some phenomenon associable with color and sex occurs in later life, increasing the risk of death from falls in females and in white persons.

Little, if any, information is available pertaining to injury rates from falls by racial group. However, studies on a small scale like that of Michael Gyepes and others suggest that Negroes suffer fewer hip fractures than do whites.[36] This has not yet been explained; but osteoporosis, which may predispose fractures, is believed to be more prevalent among the white populace than the nonwhite.

Foreign-born white persons have four times the fall death rate of native-born whites. Rates for the foreign-born are higher than for the native-born in all age groups, but the differences are greatest in children (particularly under five) and in the elderly (see Appendix Table 12).

The National Health Survey reports that almost 60 percent of fall injuries occur in the home, 11 percent on streets and highways, 9 percent in schools, and 8 percent in industrial places. About 60 percent of falls at home occur inside the house—that is, in any room, attic, or cellar or on a porch or steps leading to an entrance; the remainder occur in such places as the yard, gardens, or garage, or on the patio, driveway, or walks.

Certain types of home falls have received attention from researchers. Miller and Esmay have conducted a study of stairway falls which shows that the greatest number occur in mid-morning, mid-afternoon, and early evening. The first two periods are those in which the housewife is at the peak of her indoor activity, often carrying bundles of wash, trash, and cleaning supplies up and down stairways. The evening peak occurs at a time when the greatest number of family members are ordinarily at home—and this is a time when the number of falls by males and females is about equal.

Several other findings of the Miller and Esmay study follow: there is very little correlation between slopes of stairways and the number of falls that occur on them; no more falls occur on stairways with landings than on those without them; no more falls occur on those with winding turns than on other types of stairs; slipping is responsible for twice as many falls as any other single cause; the leading contributing factors are hurrying and having one's arms full; and twice as many slipping falls occur where there are rubber mats as where steps are merely painted (possibly due to worn conditions of the mats). In the study, 75 percent of the stairways were not uniform in treads or risers or both; 56 percent were inadequately lighted.[37]

Age-adjusted death rates for falls are highest in New England and the Middle Atlantic states; the lowest rates are in the West South

Central area. The District of Columbia (14 per 100,000 persons) and Massachusetts (12) have the highest age-adjusted rates for falls; Hawaii (4) and Mississippi (4.7) have the lowest. (See Appendix Table 29.) New England has the highest age-adjusted rate for aged persons, largely because the Massachusetts rate far exceeds any other; but several individual states—particularly Ohio and Indiana—have rates higher than the second highest state in the New England division. Lowest rates are in the West South Central division (see Appendix Table 30).

The reason for the high Massachusetts death rates for falls in elderly white persons, particularly white females, is not apparent. Comparison with the rates of other New England states would seem to eliminate weather as an important factor. However, the combination of weather conditions, high degree of urbanization, and higher proportion of white foreign-born persons than in other New England states is perhaps a partial explanation.

Both injury and death rates for falls are higher for persons living in urban areas than in rural areas, and farm dwellers have the lowest rates. However, there is little difference between urban and rural dwellers for falls in the home except for those in the rural farm home, where the rates are appreciably lower. Various studies suggest that poor housing conditions in the core city account for the higher metropolitan rates. Investigators often notice rickety step construction, lack of adequate stairway treads, dim lighting, and clutter. Data from the National Health Survey show that falls on stairs, steps, or from a height are highest in the lowest income group.

Deaths from falls are not evenly distributed over the year: the months from April through September have the lowest number of deaths and the winter months, particularly December and January, the highest (see Appendix Table 15). Variations by age and type of fall probably reflect climatic conditions—ice on outside steps and walks has been identified as a factor in wintertime falls in northern areas by Division of Accident Prevention studies—as well as sociological factors like housing, transportation, and living habits. Northern sections of the country having winters with frequent freezes and thaws generally reflect higher age-adjusted injury and death rates from falls; many of these areas, such as Massachusetts, are also urbanized. Deaths caused by falling from one level to another occur most frequently during the summer months; deaths from falls on a single level occur most frequently during the winter months. In children and young adults, deaths from falls occur most frequently during the summer and early autumn, but among the aged they are most frequent during the winter months.

The death rate for falls decreased from about 14 per 100,000 persons in 1950 to about 10 in 1963, partly because of changes in methods of classification. The seventh revision of the International Classification of Diseases, for example, transferred deaths caused by accidental falls to various categories in the disease classification and also changed the interpretation of self-inflicted injury.[38] Nevertheless, there appears to have been a genuine decline in the rates for white females, particularly in the older groups.

Falling or projected objects

Blows from falling or projected objects cause about 1,400 deaths each year—a rate of 0.8 per 100,000 persons (see Appendix Table 10). The rate is much higher in males than in females. The National Health Survey reports that each year about 4,000,000 people are injured when struck by a moving object—a rate of 23.3 per 1,000; in this category the male rate is almost three times that for females. About 40 percent of these injuries occur in the home and about 30 percent in industrial places. Such injuries account for over 13 percent of all cases of compensable work injuries.[39]

Machinery

Each year machinery accidents cause about 2,000 deaths—a rate of 1.1 per 100,000 persons (see Appendix Table 10), and injuries to more than 1,300,000 persons at the rate of 7.4 per 1,000. Of the injuries sustained from machinery in operation, almost 50 percent involve restricted activity; less than 10 percent are bed-disabling. Of impairments due to injury, 11.6 percent (1,200,000) are attributed to this type of accident; such impairments are incurred frequently by each age group, ranging from 10.4 percent at ages 15-44 to 13.4 percent at ages 45-64 (National Health Survey).

Accidents involving machinery in operation are the third highest cause of injuries (13.9 percent of all causes) leading to orthopedic impairments described as those of the "upper extremity and shoulder." Accidents involving nonmotor vehicles or machinery in operation are the leading cause of impairments described as "absence of major extremities" and "absence of fingers or toes" (39.3 percent and 53.4 percent, respectively). Such impairments are also high in work accidents: 59.0 percent for major extremities and 67.5 for fingers and toes.

Death and injury rates for machinery are, as one might guess, much higher for males than for females. Mortality from machinery accidents rises steadily from childhood through the main working years. The death rate among males increases from less than 1.0 per 100,000 persons at ages under 15 to a peak of 4.0 at ages 55-64; it decreases thereafter but remains higher, for the most part, than in early adult life. The female death rate is low at all ages.

Injuries from accidents involving machinery in operation occur most frequently among persons in age groups over 24: the 25-44 ranks first and the 65 and over second with injury rates of 13.0 and 11.2 per 1,000, respectively (National Health Survey). The male death rate is slightly higher for whites (2.2 per 100,000) than for nonwhites (1.8), and the female rate is the same (0.1) for both whites and nonwhites. The death rate is higher for Indians (1.3) than for any other nonwhite race (see Appendix Table 10).

Almost one-half (47 percent) of all fatal injuries caused by machine accidents occur on the farm—far more than in any other place—and a large proportion of them involve tractors used as such and for power takeoff. More than one-fourth (28 percent) of the deaths from machine accidents occur on industrial places and premises (see Appendix Table 38). Almost half (46 percent) of the nonfatal injuries caused by machinery occur in industrial places; the home ranks second with 36 percent. The injury rate is 2.7 per 1,000 for this type of accident occurring in the home and is about equal whether inside or outside the home (1.2 and 1.4, respectively). Males have four times the rate for females for home injuries (4.3 as opposed to 1.1). Injury rates are higher with age: 2.8 at 15-44 years and 3.6 at 65 and over.

Machinery accidents are responsible for 6.9 percent of impairments due to injury in the home, and they cause one-tenth of the impairments to the "upper extremity and shoulder." Machinery in operation causes 27 percent of the impairments due to injury while at work; it also causes 32 percent of "upper extremity and shoulder" impairments and 8.3 percent of "lower extremity and hip" impairments.

Accident death rates for machinery accidents are highest in the West North Central (2.3 per 100,000 persons) and Mountain (1.8) areas and lowest in the New England (0.5) and Middle Atlantic (0.6) divisions. (See Appendix Table 9.) Wyoming has the highest death rate (4.0) for machinery accidents and Rhode Island and the District of Columbia the lowest (0.2 for each).

Injury rates are higher among persons living in rural farm areas (8.5 per 1,000) than among those who live in either rural nonfarm (7.5) or urban (7.2) areas. Home injuries in rural nonfarm areas are at the rate of 3.9 per 1,000, compared with 2.5 in urban areas.

Over one-half (51.3 percent) of fatal machinery accidents occur during the summer months (May through September). The lowest number of fatal accidents occur in January (4.6 percent).

The death rates are slightly lower now than in the first quarter of this century, although there has been little variation from year to year. After 1940 the rates ranged from 0.8 per 100,000 during 1946-1948 to 1.4 in 1953; and after 1953 the rate decreased slightly to 1.0 in 1962-1963.

Local reports support the conclusion from National Health Survey figures that machinery in operation is the leading cause of the impairments "absence of major extremities" and "absence of fingers or toes." In a recent study of amputations in Iowa by the Division of Accident Prevention and the State University of Iowa Institute of Agricultural Medicine, investigations revealed that most of the amputations were caused while the persons injured were making mechanical adjustments to or clearing objects from machinery in operation.

In another Division study, the roles of signaling and visibility in the causation of accidents involving tractors on highways was established. (It should be noted that deaths from this type of accident are classified as motor-vehicle fatalities.) Steps are being taken to improve the lighting and signal systems of tractor on highways and their visibility to others. It was also learned that the tractor operator reacts in an emergency situation as if he were driving an automobile; as a result, tractor controls are being redesigned for similarity to corresponding automobile controls. Another study, of accidents involving tractors at work on the farm, disclosed that the largest single cause of death among those studied was the absence of appropriate protection to the operator—roll bars or crushproof containers, for example—that would increase the chance of survival in case of overturning.

Other studies, in which the Division of Accident Prevention of the Public Health Service has participated, have highlighted the circumstances surrounding specific types of machinery accidents. Findings reveal that injuries associated with rotary power lawn mowers are caused mostly by objects thrown by the mower (including parts of the mower itself), when attempts are made to adjust the motor while it is running, and when the mower is pulled backward over the foot. The investigations indicate that reel mowers are an infrequent source of accidental injury.

The problem of injuries from washing-machine wringers has been re-established through epidemiologic investigations. Wringer injuries are primarily the problem of children, particularly helpful and curious little boys. The need for more efficient safety releases on these machines was evident in many of the investigations.

Cutting and piercing instruments

Over a hundred persons are killed each year by cutting and piercing instruments (other than machinery)—a rate of about 0.1 per 100,000; most of them are males. However, about 2,700,000 persons are injured each year by such instruments, at the rate of about 15 per 1,000 (National Health Survey). Persons in the 15-24 age group have the highest injury rate, and the rate for males is about twice that for females. About 10 percent of amputations of fingers and toes are caused by such instruments. Over 50 percent of the injuries occur in or around the home and about 20 percent in industrial places. The injury rate is highest in rural nonfarm areas.

Electric current

Approximately 1,000 persons die from electric current each year in the United States, at a rate of 0.6 per 100,000, and the majority of them are males. Data on the frequency of nonfatal injuries from electricity are not available, although severe injuries, many of which involve amputation, do occur.

The death rate for children under 15 is 0.2 per 100,000; for ages 15-24, 0.8; and for 25-34, 1.1 (the highest rate in any age group). In each group thereafter the rate decreases. White persons (0.6) have a higher death rate than nonwhites (0.4). (See Appendix Table 10.)

The home area is the scene of over one-fourth of electrical deaths; about one-fifth occur in industrial places or on their premises. A Division of Accident Prevention study conducted in one northeastern city indicated that one-third of the electric-current injuries observed happened in the home (80 percent of which were in the kitchen).

However, as the preponderance among 25-34 year old males would indicate, most deaths from electric current result from injuries sustained at work but not in an industrial place. A special study of a sample of death certificates for 1957 showed that the category of work injuries having the largest number of deaths (15 percent) involved contact between the booms of cranes or similar machines and high tension wires. (Other contact in working with high-voltage lines accounted for an additional 30 percent of the deaths.) Although the subjects of this study who were killed included helpers and other workers, about 12 percent were linemen and another 12 percent electricians. Electrical tools and equipment, household appliances, and habits of play accounted for most electrical injuries at home.[40] Work with outside television antennae and the use of electrical equipment in the bathroom were revealed as common causes of death at home in a study by the Division of Accident Prevention.

Over one-half of the deaths from electric current occur during the summer months (June through September), whereas less than 17 percent occur during the winter months (November through February). (See Appendix Table 15.) The higher mortality in summer is largely the result of increased activity in the repair and extension of electrical lines as well as the greater amount of outdoor work than in winter that brings men, in particular, into accidental contact with electrical lines. The fact that perspiration lowers resistance to electric shock is also a contributing factor.

Although residential and industrial consumption of electricity has increased over the years, the death rate from accidents involving electric current has decreased. An increase has occurred simultaneously in home accidents involving electricity that is attributable to do-it-yourself activities.[41]

Burns and other injuries from fires and explosions

Accidental injuries involving burns are usually acquired in one of two ways: by involvement in an uncontrolled fire or explosion or through contact of some part of the body with a hot object, liquid, acid, or other substance or with a flame. The former is the more common cause of death and the latter of nonfatal injury. These accidents will, accordingly, be considered in two sections. (Other burns, often fatal, are from accidents involving motor vehicles, water transport, and other factors; they are classified in categories corresponding to their causes. On the other hand, some deaths and injuries are from asphyxia, fractures, and so on—with the underlying cause of fire or explosion.)

Fires and explosions of combustible materials. Fires and explosions are the third leading cause of accidental death in the United States (there are about 7,200 such deaths annually); this death rate is 4.0 per 100,000 persons (see Appendix Table 10). They are the leading cause of death from nontransport accidents to children 1-4 years old and the second leading cause to children 5-14 and persons 45 and over.

Injuries from fires are not relatively numerous but they are frequently fatal or impairing. The National Health Survey estimates that about 260,000 persons are injured each year from these causes—a rate of 1.5 per 1,000. Of the injuries sustained, nearly 75 percent result in restricted activity and about 45 percent are bed-disabling. There are about 270,000 persons with impairments due to uncontrolled fires or explosions in the United States (National Health Survey).

As can be seen in Chart 4.2, the death rate for these accidents is high for children under 5 (6.5 per 100,000), low at ages 15-24 (1.3), and highest (having risen gradually after age 24) at 85 and over (31.0). The injury rate for uncontrolled fires and explosions is highest for persons 15-24 and lowest for persons under 15 or for persons 65 and older. The National Health Survey and local sources show injury rates lowest in the young and old. This pattern is the inverse of the mortality pattern and probably indicates either the fragility of the very young and the very old or that less severe injuries are sustained by adults under 65.

The death rate for nonwhite persons (10.7 per 100,000) is more than three times the rate for white persons (3.2); the excess is prevalent everywhere in the United States and is greatest at ages under five. Under one, the rate for nonwhites (25.7) is more than seven times the rate for whites (3.5). (See Appendix Table 31.)

At practically all ages, among both white and nonwhite persons, the death rate is higher for males than for females. However, in children 5-14 the rate is higher for girls and among nonwhites in that group the rate for girls (8.7 per 100,000) is almost twice as high as that for boys (4.4). (See Appendix Table 31.) Data on injuries show higher rates for males than for females.

The death rate is higher for Indians (12.6 per 100,000) than for any other nonwhite race, and the Negro rate is the second highest (11.1). Japanese (0.9) and Chinese (1.1) have the lowest rates (see Appendix Table 13).

Among the white foreign-born the death rate (4.6 per 100,000) is greater than that of the native-born (3.0). Foreign-born persons have higher rates than do natives primarily among the very young (see Appendix Table 12). In adults, however, the rate is higher among the native-born, resulting in a higher age-adjusted rate for natives. In the South Atlantic and East South Central areas the native-born white rate is higher than that of the foreign born; but this is not true of the West South Central division.

Accident death rates for fires and explosions are highest in the East

South Central (6.8 per 100,000), West South Central (5.9), and South Atlantic (5.3) geographic divisions; rates are about equal among all other divisions. Most of the reasons for the variety of rates probably pertain to social and economic conditions: the use and misuse of flammable liquids in southern areas, for example, contributes to the high rates there. Statewise, Alaska has the highest rate (13.0) and Mississippi (10.2) the next highest (see Appendix Table 9).

The rate is higher in nonmetropolitan than in metropolitan counties (see Appendix Table 11). The absence of fire departments in non-metropolitan areas, and the use of local rather than central heating, may account for part of this excess; it is also possible that medical attention, including emergency medical services, is not as readily available in rural areas.

More than 80 percent of these deaths occur in the home. Industrial places (about 4 percent) are next highest (see Appendix Table 38). Of injuries from such accidents, about 35 percent occur in the home or on home premises, and 43 percent in industrial places.

Over half of fire and explosion deaths occur during the months of December through March (Appendix Table 15). This is especially true for deaths among the very young and the very old that occur indoors. Summer is the peak for deaths among other age groups.

Because of changes in classification and coding procedures it is difficult to determine trends in these death rates in the United States. No significant decreases are apparent in recent years, however.

Obviously, socioeconomic conditions play an important role in the occurrence of fires and explosions. Poor housing, poor safety habits, and lack of knowledge about electrical wiring systems and flammable liquids (all of which derive from other social factors) are only part of the complex problem.

Deaths and injuries from fires and explosions are usually caused by one of the following: (1) Fire originating from cooking or heating sources. (2) Smoking and the use of matches. (3) Electrical deficiencies or improper use of electrical equipment or utilities. (4) Fire in rubbish or trash. (5) Flammable liquids or gases.[42]

Fire from a defective stove frequently leads to destruction of a house or part of it and is a common cause of death—very often by entrapment—to the old and young. Defective heating equipment, particularly in stoves using petroleum products that drip or leak, is a conspicuous cause of fires in southern areas.

Smoking in bed or in overstuffed furniture is a common cause of accidental death to adults: smoking combined with drinking and falling asleep is deadly. It is estimated that smoking accounts for about 20 percent of deaths from fires in the home. Playing with matches is a common cause of burns to children, especially boys.

Defective electrical equipment, often in combination with dilapidated housing, is a frequent cause of fires. Defective wiring or switches that have not been repaired, overloaded circuits, use of the wrong fuse or of a penny in lieu of a fuse, and misuse of extension cords, contribute to the toll of deaths and injuries from fires. An entire building is often involved in such fires.

The use (and misuse) of flammable or volatile liquids contribute to the problem in many ways. Leakage from defective stoves, as mentioned above, is a common cause of home fires. Use of such liquids as starters or boosters for fires either indoors or outdoors is often the cause of conflagrations, deaths that result from clothing catching fire, and localized burns.

Purposeful setting of fires that cause death or injury is reported among children with speech, hearing, and learning disabilities. A large number of these children can be described as impulsive or poorly adjusted or both.[43]

Injuries caused by hot substances, corrosive substances, steam, or open flames. This type of accident results in only about 400 deaths per year, essentially among preschool children and elderly persons; such deaths are rare among teenagers or adults under 65. Rates are somewhat higher for nonwhites than for whites and they differ slightly from state to state although numbers are small. Approximately three-fourths of the deaths from this cause occur in the home.

Each year 1,300,000 persons are injured by contact with hot objects, open flames, and the like. Over 75 percent are injured in the home and another 18 percent in industrial places. The female injury rate (8.0 per 1,000) is higher than that of the male (7.1); the difference is more pronounced for injuries exclusively in the home, where the female rate is 7.5 compared with the male rate of 3.9. The rate of burns in the home is much higher for children than for older groups.

This accident rate is higher in urban than in rural areas and somewhat higher in rural nonfarm than in rural farm areas. Home injuries occur in rural nonfarm and urban areas at about the same rate, but the rural farm rate is somewhat lower.

Burns are universal, but the type of accident causing the burn varies with age, sex, culture, geography, weather, and other environmental or social factors including heating methods. Scalds are high in some areas and groups; and open flames are common in the South. Floor heaters frequently cause burns in some areas, especially to small children. Matches and the misuse of petroleum products are common causes of burns to boys but not to girls; climbing on stoves and reaching over lighted burners on stoves is a common problem among girls. Perhaps the greatest single hazard for burns from fires to girls is their clothing in proximity to an open flame.

Tragic incidents involve explosions of containers caused by "backflash." Ignition of gas vapors near motors by sparks from ignition systems, electrical tools, furnaces being lit, and so on are common sources of injuries to males. Females are most frequently injured while lighting stoves—sometimes allowing too much gas to flow before lighting it (ovens are often involved). Women are also injured while cleaning work clothes soaked with petroleum products or utilizing such products for the cleaning process.

Burns from trash, rubbish, or other fires are most common to men and boys, although little girls' clothing is often set on fire when they do not stay clear of flames. Explosion of pressurized metal containers burning with trash is becoming more common.

A recent study of burns to children in an urban California area showed that 24 percent of the burns were from scalds and 19 percent from floor heaters. Twenty-eight percent were to children under five.[44]

Hot liquids are a frequent cause of burns, often to women who spill or spatter grease while cooking or drop pans with hot handles. It is not uncommon for men to suffer steam burns from radiators of cars. Hot liquids are probably the most frequent cause of burns to children: coffee and water are the two leading agents. Such burns occur often when the child pulls a container of hot food or liquid from the stove, counter, or table. A very large proportion of these burns are to one-year olds. Hot water in a container on the floor (usually for cleaning purposes) or in a bathtub—sometimes accidentally turned on—is often a cause. Hot water burns are also common among very old persons, especially in homes for the aged, including nursing homes.

Burns caused by hot substances other than liquids are also incurred frequently by children. More than one-half the cases on record in the Division of Accident Prevention are to children under two, the greater number of them boys. As with liquids, such accidents occur most often in the kitchen, although the living room can also be involved. Cooking stoves, room heaters, radiators, and heat registers are common sources of burns to youngsters.

Electrical appliances are a major source of danger to small children. An electric wire, particularly one left dangling, is a temptation to a child. Pulling at the cord of a percolator or hot plate, he may be burned by the liquid contents or by the appliance itself; even a disconnected iron may still be hot enough to burn. Approximately three-fourths of all such injuries happen to children under one year of age. Another serious and not infrequent cause of injury to children is the live electric cord; serious mouth burns often result from oral contact with live extension cords.

Foreign bodies
About 2,500 people are killed each year when foreign bodies enter the eye and its adnexa or another orifice (a rate of about 1.4 per 100,000). Most of these deaths are caused by the inhalation and ingestion of food or some other object causing obstruction or suffocation. The rate is higher for males than females and for nonwhites than whites; and it is highest among Indians. The rate by age is highest for infants; it remains rather low through adulthood and increases again in persons 75 and over.

About 1,200,000 persons are injured each year by such causes—a rate of 7.0 per 1,000 (National Health Survey). The injury rate is higher for males than for females and is highest in the age group 25-44. Most injuries occur in the home or on the home premises.

Firearm accidents
Each year in the United States about 2,300 persons are accidentally killed by firearms and over 100,000 are injured. There is insufficient knowledge at present about the circumstances surrounding such deaths and injuries; but the problem is a substantial one, compounded by the large number of homicide and suicide attempts by means of firearms.

The death rate in this category is very low for children under age 1 (0.2 per 100,000); it gradually increases to a peak in the 15-24 group (2.4) and declines thereafter (see Appendix Table 36). The injury rate is quite low in each age group.

The ratio of injuries to deaths (Chart 4.5) for males indicates the seriousness of the problem in the 15-24 age group, where the ratio is quite low. The resemblance to the pattern for nonpedestrian motor vehicle accidents is striking and suggests some common factor in this age group involving increased risk-taking (playing "Russian Roulette" and "chicken," for example).

Nonwhites have a higher death rate for these accidents than do whites in all age groups (see Appendix Table 36). Among nonwhites the death rate is highest for Indians (3.6 per 100,000) and lowest for Chinese and Japanese (see Appendix Table 13). The death rate for males is about seven times that for females. The difference is particularly noticeable beginning with the 5-14 age group, for both whites and nonwhites (see Appendix Table 36). Almost all such injuries are to males.

About 14 percent of accidental firearm deaths during the period 1959-1961 occurred in places not specified on death certificates. In cases with known locations, about 56 percent occur in the home, 14 percent on the farm, and 18 percent in "other specified places"—a category that includes mountains, prairies, and other areas where people are likely to hunt with firearms. Other locations are on the street and highway (6 percent) and in public buildings (4 percent). Data concerning place of occurrence have been available since 1949. The percentage of deaths from home firearm accidents increased from 40 percent in that year to about 48 percent in 1963.

Firearm injuries occur in or around the home (30 percent), on farms (28 percent), and in the category entitled "other and unknown locations" (29 percent).

A much higher proportion of firearm deaths among women than among men occur in the home (80 percent for white females, 89 percent for nonwhite females; 50 percent for white males, 65 percent for nonwhite males).

More than 30 percent of all firearm deaths in the home happen to children under 15, and there is the least difference between the sexes in proportion of deaths in this age group. Boys have a larger proportion of deaths in the home than do older males; this is also true of nonwhites over whites. White males are more likely than nonwhite males to incur their fatal firearm accidents on farms or in "other specified places" while hunting or engaged in related activities.

Alaska has the highest death rate of the states (6.5 per 100,000 persons), followed by Mississippi (4.1) and Montana (4.0). Low rates are in Rhode Island (0.2) and in New Jersey, Massachusetts, and Connecticut (0.4 each). In general, the Mountain (2.7), East South Central (2.4), and West South Central (2.2) areas have high rates; the Middle

Atlantic (0.5) and New England (0.6) divisions have low rates. (See Appendix Table 9.)

Most firearm deaths occur in the fall and winter months, with a peak in November (14 percent). Such factors as age, sex, and color apparently do not have any appreciable effect on firearm deaths by month.

The death rate decreased from 1900 to 1964. Prior to 1940 it was 2.0 per 100,000 or higher each year (except in 1909), reaching a peak of 3.4 in 1904. From 1940 to 1964 it was 2.0 or lower each year, with the lowest rate in 1962 (1.1).

There is some indication of a relation between firearm deaths and low socioeconomic status; it is possible that urban or rural environment and geographic differences may have similar bearings. Cultural factors may also be implicated in the high death rates of males after age five. As an example, Alpenfels and Hayes cite the practice in Western societies of giving children toys that are nonfunctioning models of tools used by adults. They indict the " 'play' gun which is pointed at both the imagined and real giants of a child's world."[45]

The Missouri Department of Public Health and Welfare has published an account of the circumstances involved in 84 accidental firearm deaths in that state in 1961: 63 percent took place in the home; injuries were more often self-inflicted than inflicted by others; the head or neck and the chest were most frequently struck and together they accounted for 80 percent of the injuries; the accidents occurred more frequently on Saturdays and Sundays than on other days.[46]

During 1954-1958, the Colorado State Department of Public Health queried relatives or other respondents on circumstances under which fatal home accidents had occurred; among the deaths analyzed were 52 caused by firearms. About 85 percent of these occurred to males; about 45 percent of the victims were under 25. In about 40 percent of the cases, the type of weapon causing death was unspecified; of those specified, over one-half (19) were rifles—of which 11 were .22 caliber, and pistols (8), shotguns (5), and even a grenade (1) were mentioned. Where activities were specified, about 40 percent of the home accidents happened while a weapon was being examined or played with, about 13 percent in cleaning, repairing, or storing a weapon, and over 10 percent while loading or unloading a weapon. In approximately half of the accidents, action by a person other than the victim figured in the fatality.

The Metropolitan Life Insurance Company has reported on 79 home firearm deaths to industrial policyholders in 1956 and ordinary policy-holders in 1956-1957. In 30 percent of the cases neither activity nor circumstances was specified. Of those that were specified, the most frequent activity was preparing the weapon for use by cleaning or loading it (24 percent), followed by playing with the weapon (13 percent), playing "Russian Roulette" (9 percent), demonstrating or examining the weapon (9 percent), and pointing the weapon in jest (9 percent). In another 36 percent the activity was specified, but no single activity was frequent enough to be mentioned.[47]

In cooperation with the State Health Department, the Public Health Service recently investigated selected injuries reported by hospitals in Pennsylvania, among which were 24 cases of injuries involving firearms. Although the investigations were directed toward accidents not associated with hunting, 15 of the injuries involved hunting or target-shooting activity. All but two of the victims were males. Most of the injuries occurred in fields, woods, and other unpeopled areas, and most were self-inflicted. The majority of the victims had handled and used firearms for at least two years prior to injury; it may be misleading, therefore, to emphasize inexperience as a factor in these accidents. In several cases the weapon or the shell was found to be defective, and often the safety mechanism was weak. In many instances the foot was the injured portion of the body.

The Division of Accident Prevention, in cooperation with the Kentucky State Health Department, conducted an epidemiologic study of accidental injuries in six Appalachian counties of eastern Kentucky from June 1964 to June 1965. The reports of firearm accidents convey an intrinsic flavor of violence—of an almost "frontier" atmosphere—in the mountain culture. The accidents are related to such activities as practicing "the quick-draw," the crossing of picket lines by nonunion laborers, and the carrying of revolvers for "protection from enemies." The feeling of "need to carry a weapon" expressed by truckdrivers, and the explosive violence that seems natural to some people under intoxication, complicate the accident picture. Of the 22 cases studied, 10 involved handguns. Several of the weapons were equipped with adapted hair triggers.

The annual summaries on hunting accidents by the National Rifle Association yield useful information on how and to whom firearm accidents happen. These reports indicate that nearly all victims are males, the majority of whom have hunting licenses; about 36 percent of the victims are under 20 years of age; about 18 percent of the injuries are fatal. More than 55 percent of the injuries involve shotguns, about 35 percent rifles, and about 7 percent handguns. About 38 percent of the accidents happen while hunting small game, about 23 percent in pursuit of land birds, and about 21 percent while stalking deer.

Inexperience, mentioned earlier as a dubious factor, is sometimes blamed for firearm accidents; but it is a difficult condition to define. National Rifle Association data indicate its relative unimportance in such accidents: well over two-thirds of the shooters in Association reports have had three years or more of experience in firearm usage prior to their accidents.

In about 53 percent of these cases, the discharge of the firearm is unintentional; frequent causes include stumbling, catching the trigger on a bush or other object, inadvertently pulling the trigger, removing a weapon from or placing it in a vehicle, and crossing a fence with a loaded weapon. Data do not include information on the condition of safety mechanisms.

Reasons offered for accidental injury by intentional discharge of a weapon include: "victim out of sight of shooter," "victim covered by shooter swinging on game," or "victim mistaken for game."[48]

At one time in the history of our country firearms were important for survival; they were needed for both sustenance and defense. The right to bear arms was considered inalienable and was thus written into the United States Constitution. But cultures gradually change. Today, legitimate use of firearms is largely restricted to recreation, law enforcement, and military operations. Nevertheless, many people still attribute to them the values they had in the past; this has resulted in vehement controversies over the degree of accessibility to firearms guaranteed by the Constitution. On the one hand, firearms symbolize nontransferable individual rights; on the other hand, they represent disorder and risk, negating these rights. They signify both danger and protection. Society is left with the need to find some method of mitigating the dangers without infringing upon our ideals of freedom.

Mechanical suffocation

In 1960 approximately 1,500 persons died in the United States as a result of mechanical suffocation (0.9 per 100,000). Over 1,200 of the deaths were to infants—a rate of 29.6 or about 30 percent of all accidental deaths to children under one. Mechanical suffocation in bed and cradle is the leading cause of accidental death in this group;

in fact, 60 percent of these deaths are to children one through three months old.

The death rate was higher in 1960 for nonwhites than for whites, especially for suffocation in bed or cradle. Rates were generally higher for males than for females. Nearly 80 percent of the deaths occurred in the home, and among infants 84 percent occurred in bed or cradle.

The southern areas have the highest infant death rates for mechanical suffocation in bed or cradle, the East South Central area having 44 per 100,000 persons, the South Atlantic 38, and the West South Central 28. New England has the lowest rate, 17. Nonmetropolitan counties have rates twice as high as do metropolitan counties (37 and 18, respectively, per 100,000). Over 50 percent of these deaths occur during the months of November through March.

The death rate for mechanical suffocation in bed or cradle underwent a gradual decline after 1949, reaching a level in 1963 about one-half that of 1949. This is true of the total rate and of the infant rate. Mechanical suffocation other than in bed or cradle stayed at about the same level during this period.

In 1959, it became apparent that plastics—especially plastic film used by dry-cleaning and other industries—were causing deaths to children by suffocation. By arrangement with the Division of Vital Statistics, the Division of Accident Prevention reviewed the death certificates for victims of mechanical suffocation involving plastics at the outset of a nationwide information campaign. The latter division then reviewed the deaths from the same cause in 1961, following a year of extensive public education. The infant rate alone was 40 percent lower in 1961 than it had been in 1959 (4.2 to 2.5 per 100,000). The reduction appeared in each color-sex group.

In recent years the subject of accidental mechanical suffocation, which often involves infants who are discovered dead in their beds or cradles, has provoked many studies and articles. The general thesis of much of this literature is that deaths are often attributed to mechanical suffocation when the actual cause is a suddenly acute disease condition. It is widely recommended that in each case of suspected mechanical suffocation of an infant an autopsy be performed.

It may be partly as a result of this heavy volume of literature that deaths from mechanical suffocation, particularly in bed or cradle, appear to have decreased in recent years. (That is, deaths that might once have been so categorized may now, as a result of more sophisticated methods in pathology, be reported as deaths from infection.)

Nevertheless, many deaths of children still occur in discarded refrigerators, washing machines, and the like.

Animals and insects

About 200 people are killed each year by animals and insects; about 60 of them die from bites and stings. About three-quarters of the victims are males. Farms and homes are the locations of most of these deaths.

Almost 2,000,000 persons receive injuries annually from this cause— a rate of 10.4 per 1,000 (National Health Survey). The rate is somewhat higher in males than in females (12.7 and 8.2, respectively); children under 15 have the highest rate for any age group, and the rate decreases with age. The rate is highest in rural nonfarm areas, second highest on rural farms, and lowest in urban areas; three-fourths of the injuries occur in the home. Reporting systems instituted by the Division of Accident Prevention suggest that at least half of these injuries are from dog bites, with cat bites less frequent; rat bites are still existent, expecially in cities. Dogs bite legs and hands most frequently, but in preschool children some serious head injuries have been noted.

A study by Henry Parrish and others of snakebites states that approximately 7,000 persons in the United States are bitten by poisonous snakes annually. Rates are highest among children in the 5-19 group, higher in males than in females, and higher among whites than nonwhites. Ninety-five percent of snakebites occur from April through October.[49]

In places where animal research is conducted, injuries caused by animals are frequent.

Other causes

Another type of accident that causes death is the explosion of pressure vessels; and excessive heat or cold, hunger, thirst, exposure, and radiation are further causes of death.

About 150 persons are killed by lightning each year in the United States, the majority in summer. Of the 129 deaths due to lightning in 1960, 53 occurred on farm premises (excluding farm homes), 20 in the home, 14 in places of recreation and sport, 5 on streets and highways, 4 in public buildings, and 33 in other and unspecified places.[50]

Tornadoes, hurricanes, and floods claimed 524 lives in the United

States (with the exception of Alaska and Hawaii) during the five years 1959-1963. Tornadoes accounted for 214 of the deaths, floods 184, and hurricanes 126. Floods and tornadoes, as a rule, claim their largest tolls during spring and early summer, hurricanes generally in late summer and early autumn.[51]

There are several major causes of injury, according to the National Health Survey, not included in the classification of deaths. Some of these follow.

About 3,500,000 injuries are caused each year when people bump into objects or other people—a rate of 19.8 per 1,000 persons. The rate is about twice as high for males as for females, and it is highest among persons in the age group 15-24; it is highest, too, in urban areas.

Almost 2,000,000 people are injured each year from being caught in, pinched by, or crushed between two objects—a rate of 10.7 per 1,000. Male and female rates are about the same; the highest rate is in persons aged 65 and over and the next highest in children under 15. Rural farm areas have the highest rates and urban the lowest; and about half of the injuries occur in the home or on the home premises.

Another common cause of injury is called "one-time lifting or exertion," which produces over 2,000,000 injuries annually in the United States for a rate of 12.5 per 1,000 persons. The rate for males is about twice that for females and is highest in persons 45-64 years of age. Rural farm areas have the highest rate; and over one-third of the injuries occur in or around the home and another one-third in industrial places.

About 2,500,000 people are injured each year from handling or stepping on rough objects—a rate of 14.3 per 1,000. There is little difference in the male and female rates, but children under 15 have the highest rate for any age group. The rate is highest in rural nonfarm areas; about two-thirds of the injuries occur in or about the home.

About 1,800,000 people injure themselves each year by twisting or stumbling, for a rate of 10.2 per 1,000. The rate is higher for males than for females; it is highest for persons 15-24. About 40 percent of the injuries occur in or around the home and about 15 percent in school areas; the rate is higher in urban than in rural areas.

About 1,400,000 people have injuries described as "therapeutic misadventures" (when a surgeon's knife slips or an incorrect drug dosage is administered, for example); here the rate is somewhat higher for the male than for the female, and it is highest among children under 15.

5 / ENVIRONMENTAL FACTORS

In a general sense, one's environment includes not only physical setting but, also, aspects of the culture to which one belongs. Social and cultural factors of accident causation have already been discussed in Chapter 3, "Host Factors"; discussions in this chapter will be limited to factors of time and place. It should be emphasized, however, that because environment cannot be considered apart from the host and agent, much of the discussion relating to it has been included in Chapter 4, "Agent or Type of Accident."

Home

Accidents in or about the home cause over one-half of all nontransport accidental deaths (see Appendix Table 38). The home and its premises are the scene of over half of all accidental deaths to children under five and about 40 percent of such deaths to the aged.

About 85 percent of all deaths from fires and explosions occur in the home; the highest proportions of these deaths are in the preschool child and the aged. About 85 percent of poisoning deaths by solid or liquid substances occur there; the proportions are much higher in preschool children than in adults. About 70 percent of deaths from gaseous vapors occur at home; the percentages are highest in the preschool child and in older persons. About 65 percent of deaths from falls occur there, with proportions highest among infants, preschool children, and older persons.

About 10 percent of drownings occur in the home or on home premises. Nearly all infant drownings occur at home, but practically none of the drownings in the 15-24 age group do; later, the proportion increases with advancing age.

Over one-half (56 percent) of deaths from firearms occur at home or on home premises; as might be expected, the highest percentage is in preschool children and in persons over 84. However, it is interesting that in every age group over half of these deaths occur in the home, with the exception of the 15-24 age group, in which the proportion is somewhat less than half. More detail on such accidents can be found in the section of Chapter 4 entitled "Firearm Accidents."

Of all deaths from nontransport accidents, the proportion occurring in the home is somewhat higher for nonwhite persons (63 percent) than for white persons (55 percent). The proportion for females (75 percent) is higher than that for males (45 percent). Among children under five, the percentage is about 86.

Two-thirds of all accidental deaths in the home occur to the aged and to children under five (44 and 21 percent respectively).

The proportion of nontransport accident deaths occurring in the home is highest in the East North Central, Middle Atlantic, and South Atlantic geographic divisions, and lowest in the Mountain States. The proportion of deaths from fires and explosions that occur at home is highest in the South Atlantic division and second highest in the East North Central division; lowest is the Mountain area.

About 19,000,000 persons are injured in or about the home each year (National Health Survey)—roughly 45 percent of all persons injured. The rate is 106.5 per 1,000 persons, and it is somewhat higher for males (114.0) than for females (98.5). (See Appendix Table 46.) About 53 percent of the injuries happen inside the home; in this category the percentage of male accidental injuries is about 45 percent and that for females 60 percent. Preschool children and aged persons have the highest home injury rates, and the lowest rate is in the age group 15-24. Among children boys have higher rates than girls, but among the aged women have much higher rates than men.

The injury rate among persons living in rural nonfarm areas (125.6 per 1,000) exceeds that among those who live in urban (109.9) or rural farm (111.6) areas. This higher rate applies to both males and females. The injury rate outside the house, however, is highest in rural farm areas; inside the house it is highest in urban areas (National Health Survey). The rate is somewhat higher for white persons (109.7 per 1,000) than for nonwhites (81.9). (See Appendix Table 46.)

About 34 percent of all persons injured in home accidents are injured in falls, for which, as mentioned earlier, the rate is higher than for any other accident type. The injury rate from falls is higher for females than for males. On the other hand, the rates from machinery in operation and from cutting and piercing instruments are higher for males than for females.

The home injury rate is lowest for persons in the family income group under $2,000 annually and highest in the income group $2,000-$3,999 (National Health Survey). Bed-disability days, however, are highest in the income group under $2,000; this may reflect either more serious injuries incurred, longer recovery time required, or type of work performed.

Socioeconomic factors, including the influence of customs, mores, and habits, profoundly affect the type and frequency of accidents in or about the home. (In burns, for instance, methods of cooking, heating, and trash disposal, and even types of clothing worn, can play a role.) Examples are given in the section of Chapter 3 entitled "Socioeconomic Factors" and in the discussions above of particular types of accidents. As mentioned in the section on socioeconomic factors, certain elements associable with poor, dilapidated, or substandard housing greatly affect the frequency of some accidental injuries. Further, technical changes and the rapid development of labor-saving devices introduce new hazards constantly.

Data from injury reporting systems show that the yard is the most common location of home accidents, and falls and cuts the most frequent types of accident. Indoors, the kitchen is the primary location and falls, cuts, and burns from hot substances most common. The bedroom, stairs, and living room are also frequent locations and falls are the major type of accident for each.

Information gained from a Division of Vital Statistics supplement in 1952-1953 to the standard death certificate for home accidents showed that the bedroom was the main location for fatal accidents, followed by the kitchen and living room. In the bedroom the most frequent accident types were falls, fire, and mechanical suffocation, and in the kitchen and living room falls and fire were most frequent. Outside the home, accidents occurred most often on stairs and in yards.

The use of small tractors for cutting grass, removing snow, and power takeoff is a new source of home accidents in suburban areas.

Farm
About 6 percent of all nontransport accidental deaths in the United States occur on farms, not including the farm home and its premises (see Appendix Table 38). The chief cause of death on the farm is machinery—in fact, 45 percent of all machinery deaths occur on the farm. Seventy percent of all fatalities caused by animals occur on the farm; this is true for 41 percent of lightning accidents, 14 percent of accidents with firearms, 10 percent of those with electric current, and 8 percent of all drownings. Most fatalities on farms are to males; in general, death rates are highest in the age groups over 55.

The tractor is a particularly serious accident problem on the farm— when it is ridden and when it is being used for power takeoff, both. The use of a tractor as a motor vehicle on the highway is also a problem because of its slow speed and the controls peculiar to it. (This is discussed in the section "Machinery" of Chapter 4.)

Approximately 2 percent of all injuries in the United States occur on farms (again not including farm homes and their premises). As might be guessed, the percentages of both injuries and deaths are highest for firearms and machinery. Proportionately more males than females are injured on farms, and (unlike deaths) the highest proportion is in the age group 25-44.

Industrial place and premise

The National Safety Council estimates that 14,100 deaths occur each year from accidents incurred at work. This is a rate of about 20 per 100,000 workers. The rate for mining and quarrying is highest; construction and agriculture also have high rates. Low rates are in trade, manufacturing, service, and government.[1] About 3,000 of the total number of deaths are in the motor-vehicle category.[2]

Death certificates do not provide specific data for work accidents, but information can be gained from place of occurrence. About 6 percent of nontransport accidental deaths occur in industrial places and on their premises, with machinery, falls, and blows from falling or projected objects the most frequent types of accidents. Another 1.4 percent of nontransport accidental deaths occur at mines and quarries, where blows from falling or projected objects, drowning, and machinery are the leading causes of death (see Appendix Table 38).

The National Safety Council estimates that there were 2,100,000 disabling injuries from work accidents in 1965.[3] (A disabling injury is defined as one that prevents the victim from performing any of his usual activities for a full day beyond the day of the accident.[4]) The Council also estimates that 235,000,000 man-days were lost that year because of injuries (40,000,000 by injured workers and 195,000,000 by other workers).[5]

National Health Survey estimates show that there are over 8,000,000 persons injured annually while at work; over 24,000,000 bed-disability days result from these injuries.

Males have nearly seven times the injury rate of females at work; white and nonwhite rates are about the same. Bed-disability days per 1,000 population for nonwhites is twice the number for whites. Injury rates are highest for ages 25-44 and 45-64 and lowest for aged persons. Bed-disability days per 1,000 population are highest for persons 45-64 and lowest for persons 15-24. (See Appendix Tables 46 and 47.)

Lowest injury rates are among persons with annual family incomes of under $2,000 or of $7,000 and over. For bed-disability days per

1,000 population, the highest rate is among those in the income group under $2,000, decreasing to those in the $7,000 and over group (see Appendix Tables 46 and 47). Injury rates decrease according to years of education: the highest rate is among persons with 0-4 years of schooling and the lowest among the college-educated (see Appendix Table 56).

Persons in the North Central geographic region have the highest injury rates and those in the Northeast the lowest (see Appendix Table 46). The West has the highest rate of bed-disability days per 1,000 population, and North Central and Northeast the lowest (see Appendix Table 47).

The most frequent types of work injuries in industrial places are in the categories "struck by moving object," "one-time lifting or exertion," and falls. Machinery and cutting or piercing instruments are also frequent causes of accidents. In work injuries elsewhere, falls, moving motor vehicles, and cutting or piercing instruments are major causes; one-time lifting or exertion and bumping into an object or person are also important (National Health Survey).

The National Safety Council notes that between 1912 and 1965 death rates for work accidents were reduced by 67 percent.[6] Industry has begun to realize that much work time is lost as a result of injuries that occur away from the job, and many organizations are involving themselves in educational programs to lower injury rates from off-the-job accidents. The Council estimates that there were 36,200 off-the-job accidental deaths to workers in 1965; estimates are that 22,600 were from motor-vehicle accidents and 6,300 happened in the home.[7]

Place of recreation and sport
Less than 2 percent of deaths from nontransport accidents happen in places designated for recreation and sport (see Appendix Table 38). This in no way expresses the importance of such accidental deaths and injuries, because most of the activities involved take place in areas other than those specifically for sports and recreation—falls and firearm accidents, for example. Problems of home swimming pools for small children, of drowning in bodies of water other than those designated for boating and recreation, of injuries to children in school playgrounds—all draw attention to injuries in recreation. Many water accidents connected with recreation are discussed in the section "Drowning" in Chapter 4. Injuries to small children hit in the head by wooden swings, and the general problems of design of other equip-

ment used by children for sports, indicate an area that needs special study.

Hardly any sport does not have associated injuries. Of 95 fatalities directly associated with football during the years 1960-1964, 66 were to high school students.[8] Football has the particular hazard of injuries to the face and teeth; the use of headgear, mouthpieces, and other safety equipment undergoes constant evaluation.

Skiing is gaining in popularity in the United States, and it is estimated that about 50,000 persons are injured on the slopes each year. Sprains and fractures of the ankle and knee are common. In a study sponsored by the Division of Accident Prevention, it was found that beginners suffer injuries on the slopes at a much higher rate than intermediate and advanced skiers, indicating the need for instruction in the early stages of association with the sport or the use of specially designed equipment. Ankle fractures seem to be more common in females than in males, inferring lack of protection afforded by bindings: the force required to disengage ski boots from their bindings tends to exceed the energy threshold of females.[9] A study conducted in Sun Valley, Idaho, concludes that although special safety devices help prevent accidents, education, judgment, courtesy, and current information about ski-slope conditions are most important.[10]

A review of mountaineering accidents in the United States indicates that approximately 12 persons are killed and 43 injured annually. The most common cause is slipping on rocks or snow; inexperience and inadequate equipment are contributory factors.[11]

It is estimated that more than 25,000 persons drive automobiles in various types of auto racing each year. Over 150 drivers were killed in races during the period 1960-1964. An average of about 5 drivers are killed in motorcycle races each year.[12]

Resident institution

About 8 percent of all deaths from nontransport accidents occur in places described as resident institutions (see Appendix Table 38). This category includes children's homes, orphanages, dormitories, homes for the aged, hospitals, prisons, and reform schools. More than one-half of the deaths are to females; the proportion increases with age. The excess of female over male rates is particularly true for deaths from falls—the most common cause of death from accidents in institutions (see Appendix Table 38). Fires and explosions are a problem in resident institutions: serious difficulties arise in attempting to escape from a burning building, especially for older persons. There are also problems of burns other than from fires and explosions (from hot water while bathing, for example); and injuries from excessive heat and insolation are a problem to elderly persons.

Accidental injuries to patients in nursing homes for the aged present a particular problem. In a study carried out by the Division of Accident Prevention and the Pennsylvania State Health Department it was determined that falls are the most common injury-causing accident in such homes. Falls that occur while getting into or out of bed, a chair, or a wheel chair—or while seated in the latter—are most common. Falls that occur while walking on wet surfaces and while getting on or off a commode, as well as those caused by dizziness or loss of consciousness and many that are unexplained, were encountered during the study. It was learned that, as might be expected, many fractured hips occur without obvious reasons for the falls that cause them. (This was discussed in the section "Falls" in Chapter 4.) A common type of accident in nursing homes is bumping into things, often by going through swinging doors with no window or other method of viewing the area behind the doors. Burns from hot liquids are also sustained frequently.

A major problem is the failure of patients to lock their wheel chairs before attempting to get into or out of the chairs. Another problem, of recent development, involves lightweight plastic chairs used in dining rooms, bedrooms, and lounges: although they are relatively inexpensive and easy to clean, they tend to be slippery and to provide insufficient support to patients who lean on them.

Accidental injuries in general hospitals are of two kinds: those to patients and those to hospital employees. Injuries to patients are a function of the characteristics of patients and the conditions for which the patients are admitted. Falls are the main problem here as in other resident institutions; but among newborn infants suffocation is a particular problem. Further, incorrect medication or treatment is quite common.

In one study of injuries to hospital employees the following factors were identified: puncture wounds from needles; lacerations from broken glass; burns from hot liquids, autoclaves, and acids; and strains and sprains of the back caused by lifting heavy objects. However, as in any other institution, injuries from falls were among the most serious, exceeded only by those from lifting.[13]

Accidental injuries and deaths occur in all types of resident institutions. In general, the frequency and types of accidents reflect the kind of institution involved and the composition of its population.

Geography

Alaska has the highest death rate from accidents among the states (see Appendix Table 9). The geographic distribution of accidental deaths is a function not only of accident type, but also of the age, sex, color, and other characteristics of the people who live in the area under consideration. For all accidents, the Mountain division has the highest death rates and Middle Atlantic and New England divisions the lowest. Alaska has the highest rates for fires and explosions, firearms, and drowning. New England has the highest rate for falls; motor-vehicle death rates are highest in the Mountain states.

The injury rate is highest in the West and lowest in the Northeast (see Appendix Table 59). The higher rate in the West appears to be valid for all age groups under 65. Rates for persons under 25 appear to be lowest in the South but rates for the aged highest. The geographic distribution of deaths and injuries for particular types of accidents is discussed in the section for each type of accident in Chapter 4.

Season and weather

The time of year in which accidents occur is related to the type of accident and to the age, sex, and other characteristics of the persons injured or killed. In general, deaths tend to be high in the winter, especially for old people; injuries from falls and other accidents to the elderly are also higher then. Children of school age have their highest injury and death rates in the summer, during vacations from school; at that time they are exposed to more hazards, and the range of their activities is greatest and their supervision often least. Obviously, deaths from drowning and other summer sports are higher in all persons during the summer. Season is discussed further above, under each particular type of accident.

In addition to the direct effect on accident potential of winter (in terms of ice, fog, rain, and so on), changes in weather conditions may have an effect on people's moods, reaction speeds, working efficiency, and, therefore, accidents.

The traditional approach to accident prevention has been through the study of causal factors classified by external cause in the E-code of the International Classification of Diseases. This code categorizes type of accident according to agent (motor vehicle, fire) involved and action (fall, submersion) resulting in injury or death. In order to institute emergency medical services, organize treatment facilities, and carry out secondary prevention programs it is necessary to have some knowledge of the nature of injuries and their relationship to type of accident; the International Classification also includes a code for nature of injury (N-code).

It is estimated that in the period July 1964-June 1965, 54,000,000 nonfatally injured persons sustained over 56,000,000 injuries. About 5 percent received more than one injury serious enough to require medical care or to restrict activity. The most complete statistics on the nature of such injuries are given for the period 1957-1961, in a publication of the National Center for Health Statistics.[1] Table 6.1, derived from that source, shows the percentage distribution of injuries according to type.

Of the injuries occurring in any particular year, about 33 percent are described as lacerations, 17 percent as contusions, 8 percent as fractures, and 5 percent as head injuries, including skull fractures and other injuries described in Table 6.1. Unpublished material from the National Health Survey shows that, when particular types of accidents are considered, the highest proportions of head injuries are from accidents involving moving motor vehicles and falls from a height. (This includes only skull fractures and injuries to the scalp that may involve brain damage: N-code numbers, N800, N801, N803, and N850-N856.) Other fractures result mainly from falls, with moving motor-vehicle accidents second. One-time lifting or exertion accounts for most strains and sprains of the back, but about one-fifth of these injuries occur in moving motor-vehicle accidents. Most burns occur in accidents involving hot objects or an open flame.

Data from reporting systems involving injured persons treated in hospitals correspond with data from the National Health Survey in regard to head injuries and fractures due to motor-vehicle accidents and falls, and regarding certain statistics on burns and amputations. Activities involving sports are frequently mentioned in fracture cases among young people. One injury that often occurs in sports—especially

Table 6.1   Percent distribution of current injuries by type of injury,
            separately for males and females: United States,
            July 1957-June 1961

Type of injury	Both sexes	Male	Female
All injuries	100.0	100.0	100.0
Skull fractures and head injury, n.e.c.	4.8	5.5	3.8
Other fractures and dislocations	9.4	8.9	10.0
Fracture of femur	0.3	*	*
Other fractures	7.3	7.1	7.6
Dislocations	1.8	1.7	1.9
Sprains and strains of back	5.3	5.3	5.3
Other sprains and strains	12.3	11.7	13.0
Lacerations and abrasions	31.3	34.5	27.0
Contusions	17.2	14.8	20.5
Burns	4.1	3.9	4.4
Adverse effects of medical/surgical procedures	4.6	3.5	6.0
All other current injuries	11.1	11.9	10.0
Poisonings	1.7	1.9	1.5
Other current injuries	9.3	10.0	8.5

Note: n.e.c. = not elsewhere classified.

Source: Types of Injuries, Incidence and Associated Disability:
         United States, July 1957-June 1961 (National Center for Health
         Statistics: Washington, April 1964), Series 10-No. 8, table B.

football—is fracture of the jaw, including the fracture of teeth; motor-vehicle accidents are also a major factor in such injuries. About two-thirds of all burns involve hot substances, and one-third fire and explosion. Most amputations are caused by machinery.

More than half of all nonfatal skull fractures and head injuries occur to children under 15 and incidence decreases with age. Table 6.2 shows the proportion of head injuries in a given period decreasing from 7.6 percent in the group under 15 to 2.7 in the group 45-64; further, the proportion is higher in males than in females. Other studies conducted by the Division of Accident Prevention of the Public Health Service show the same tendency of younger children to suffer head injuries: if an injury occurs, the younger the child the greater the probability of injury to the head. These studies show that about one-quarter of all treated injuries in children are to the head, about one-third to the arm, and about one-quarter to the leg; about

Table 6.2 Percent distribution of average annual number of current injuries by age, sex, and type of injury: United States, July 1957-June 1961

Type of injury; sex	All ages	Under 15	15-24	25-44	45-64	65+
Both Sexes						
All injuries	100.0	100.0	100.0	100.0	100.0	100.0
Skull fractures and head injury, n.e.c.	4.8	7.6	4.0	2.8	2.7	*
Other fractures and dislocations	9.4	5.7	9.5	10.8	12.0	16.5
Sprains and strains of back	5.3	1.1	5.7	7.7	10.2	5.4
Other sprains and strains	12.3	7.6	16.5	13.3	15.6	15.1
Lacerations and abrasions	31.3	42.1	28.6	29.1	21.5	13.5
Contusions	17.2	13.2	20.0	16.9	18.7	29.8
Burns	4.1	3.5	3.8	5.2	4.4	*
Adverse effects of medical/surgical procedures	4.6	7.7	2.2	2.9	3.6	*
All other current injuries	11.1	11.6	9.6	11.2	11.3	10.2
Male						
All injuries	100.0	100.0	100.0	100.0	100.0	100.0
Skull fractures and head injury, n.e.c.	5.5	8.8	4.6	3.5	*	*
Other fractures and dislocations	8.9	5.5	10.0	10.8	10.9	17.2
Sprains and strains of back	5.3	*	4.5	8.3	10.6	*
Other sprains and strains	11.7	7.1	17.9	12.4	14.2	*
Lacerations and abrasions	34.5	45.1	28.2	29.7	26.6	23.3
Contusions	14.8	12.0	18.4	15.8	15.3	17.9
Burns	3.9	3.2	4.8	4.2	4.3	*
Adverse effects of medical/surgical procedures	3.5	6.1	*	*	*	*
All other current injuries	11.8	11.2	9.9	13.5	12.8	*
Female						
All injuries	100.0	100.0	100.0	100.0	100.0	100.0
Skull fractures and head injury, n.e.c.	3.8	5.7	*	*	*	*
Other fractures and dislocations	10.0	6.0	8.6	10.8	13.2	16.2
Sprains and strains of back	5.3	*	8.2	6.9	9.7	*
Other sprains and strains	13.0	8.4	13.6	14.7	17.2	15.7
Lacerations and abrasions	27.0	37.6	29.4	28.2	16.1	8.9
Contusions	20.5	15.1	23.3	18.4	22.4	35.3
Burns	4.4	4.0	*	6.7	4.5	*
Adverse effects of medical/surgical procedures	6.0	10.1	*	4.6	4.3	*
All other current injuries	10.0	12.1	9.2	7.8	9.6	9.2

Note: n.e.c. = not elsewhere classified.

Source: Types of Injuries, Incidence and Associated Disability: United States, July 1957-June 1961 (National Center for Health Statistics: Washington, April 1964), Series 10-No. 8, table 5.

9 percent are to the trunk, 3 percent to the shoulder, and 1 percent to the hip.

A study conducted by the Division in cooperation with the city of Worcester, Massachusetts, showed that of all injuries treated in hospitals in the reporting area the percentage of head injuries was 59 in infants, 56 in children aged 1-4, 41 in the 5-9 group, and 22 in the 10-14. Injuries to legs and arms showed the converse pattern, increasing with age from about 30 percent in children under 5 to 75 percent in children 10-14.

In a study of injuries to children treated at a group health organization in California, Dean Manheimer and others reported on nature of injury and part of the body injured. They showed that for both boys and girls the ratio of injuries above to those below the waist decreased with age.[2]

Various sources show that head injuries—particularly skull fractures—are the most common injury type in motor-vehicle fatalities. A quite complete account of the nature of injuries sustained in passenger motor-vehicle accidents, investigated in conjunction with the Cornell Crash Injury Project in predominantly rural areas, can be found in many of the Project's publications: in general, skull fractures are most common in males, to persons ejected from a car, to occupants of "soft-tops," and from accidents at high speeds and in the early morning hours. Of all injured occupants of passenger motor vehicles, 70 percent suffer head injuries, the leading cause of which is impact with (sometimes through) the windshield, followed by impact with the steering assembly or the instrument panel or unidentified objects within the car, and ejection.[3] Many sources show head injuries to be even more of a problem to motorcyclists than to passenger or drivers of automobiles.

Fractures other than those to the head tend to increase proportionately with age in both males and females (Table 6.2). Sprains and strains of the back also increase with age, especially in males. A relatively infrequent nonfatal injury in young persons that is a relatively frequent fatal injury in old persons is fracture of the hip or femur. (This is discussed in "Accidents to the Aged," Chapter 3, and in "Falls," Chapter 4.)

In a Division of Accident Prevention study of amputations treated in a rural area in Iowa, the finger was most often amputated; toes were second in order, amputation of which was caused most often by rotary power mowers. Other types of machines were involved in amputation of fingers, arms, and other parts of the body. Amputations (other than of toes) in this part of Iowa was the problem of middle-aged men rather than of young or very old persons, home power tools were frequently involved.

For the period July 1959-June 1961 in the United States, over 50 percent of all impairments classified as absence of fingers or toes due to injuries occurred at work, as did 40 percent of those classified as absence of major extremities.[4] The causes of most of these impairments involved machinery.

As mentioned in the section "Childhood Accidents" (Chapter 3), washing-machine wringers and bicycles are common causes of injuries to children and as such are confined almost completely to youth. Injuries caused by washing-machine wringers involve severe compressions of the hand and arm; but parents often delay seeking medical attention for their children because the injury is presumed to be a minor one. In a recent article by Berish Strauch, the bicycle-spoke injury is discussed and its similarity to that of the washing-machine wringer mentioned. In the case of the bicycle, of course, the foot is usually caught in the spokes.[5]

The Public Health Service does not classify death certificates by nature of injury; but this was done in Illinois for the period 1957-1961.[6] Although these statistics are not necessarily representative of the United States, it is interesting to note that 20 percent of all the deaths due to injury involved fractures of skull or face. Motor-vehicle accidents caused 70 percent of all the deaths involving skull fracture; and about 33 percent of fatal motor-vehicle injuries involved skull fractures. Another 14 percent of the latter involved other head injuries, and about 33 percent involved internal injuries. Data from the Cornell Project show that about 60 percent of deaths to occupants of motor vehicles are from head injuries. Fractures of lower limbs are involved in about one-half of deaths from falls and skull fractures in about one-fifth; another 14 percent involve other head injuries.

The longest period of restricted activity due to accidental injury in a given period was in cases of fracture of the femur, with averages of 58.5 disability days and 38.3 bed-disability days per injury. Second were other fractures, with averages of 18.3 days of restricted activity but only 4.5 days of bed-disability. In decreasing order for days of restricted activity were: dislocations, sprains and strains of the back, contusions, and burns;[7] the number of days was greater for males than for females in every instance except in cases of fractures of the femur and contusions.

The study of homicide in the United States has taken many directions, which leads to the conclusion that a number of social and psychological variables relate to its occurrence. Norms and customs, influence of peers, and established sex roles are but a few of the social variables which, together with attitudes and the temperament and total personality of an individual, contribute to the probability of one's becoming a homicide offender or a victim.

Lack of a set of nationwide statistics to relate data on the victim and his offender handicaps the individual researcher studying clues of circumstances surrounding homicide. Accordingly, many studies have been concerned exclusively with either the victim or the offender.

In this chapter the demographic extent of the problem, as well as some of the social variables that are believed to influence the homicide rate, will be presented through a resume of vital statistics (primarily 1959-1961 mortality data) and findings from selected literature. Statistics and studies will be of homicides recognized as homicides in which the killer has been identified; it is important to bear in mind that characteristics of killers who have not been identified may not be the same. The section "Statistics" deals with vital statistics data (E-code numbers E964 and E980-E984, including deaths from injuries inflicted by others with intent to kill or injure, not in war) on victims and observable patterns and trends in homicide that have been noted since the beginning of the century. The section "Summary of the Literature" presents salient findings on criminal homicide describing victim-offender interaction, backgrounds of offenders, and homicidal motives and methods. This information is derived from individual studies based primarily on police records and, nationally, on the annual publication *Uniform Crime Reports,* of the Federal Bureau of Investigation.

Statistics

For the period 1959-1961, a yearly average of 8,358 persons met death by homicide in the United States—an annual rate of 4.7 per 100,000 population. Of the victims, 6,183 (approximately three-fourths) were males.

Children under 15 and adults over 65 have the lowest rates as homicide victims. Rates are low at ages 5-14 (0.5 per 100,000) and higher at 15-24 (5.8); they reach a peak at 25-34 (9.4) and drop steadily thereafter, reaching a low rate after age 75 (2.6), their second lowest point. The pattern of low rates under age 15 and of increase at ages 15-24 is much more pronounced for nonwhites than for either native-born or foreign-born whites (see Appendix Table 39).

Although both white and nonwhite rates vary by age, they are proportionately higher for males than for females. The ratio of males to females is about 1 to 1 in the younger age groups, but it increases to 3 to 1 in the 15-24 group; this ratio remains fairly constant during the next two decades but rises at ages 55-74 to almost 4 to 1 then dropping at age 75 and over to 2 to 1. The ratio of nonwhite males to nonwhite females is greater than the white male-female ratio.

Homicide plays a larger role in the mortality of nonwhites than of whites in the United States. Mortality rates, from highest to lowest, for the four color-sex groups are: nonwhite males (34.0 per 100,000), nonwhite females (9.4), white males (3.6), and white females (1.5). (See Appendix Table 39.)

Homicide rates (victims) for nonwhites are over 8 times as high as for native-born whites (see Appendix Table 39). Among nonwhites, rates run much higher for the Negro than for other races, accounting for most of the difference between white and nonwhite rates. For instance, the total homicide rate for Negroes (22.6 per 100,000) is almost twice the Indian rate, which is second highest (12.9); it is over 7 times the Chinese (3.0) and 15 times the Japanese rate (1.5). For each nonwhite group the male-female ratio is about 4 to 1 with the exception of the Japanese, whose ratio is about 1 to 1. For the total United States, white foreign-born and white native-born rates are quite similar, although variations exist by geographic division (see Appendix Table 42).

Age-adjusted homicide rates are highest for divorced persons (21.5 per 100,000) and for widows and widowers (19.9); married persons (5.4) have the lowest rates (see Appendix Table 41). This general pattern holds for each color-sex group. In the female, differences between the single and the married are slight. It is interesting that among the aged the rate for widows and widowers is low (see Appendix Table 41). Also noteworthy is the fact that single persons under 20 have the lowest age specific rate, as was the case with accidents.

According to the National Center for Health Statistics, standardized mortality ratios for homicide in 1950 for males aged 20-64 were highest for laborers and agricultural workers and lowest for professional, clerical, and sales workers.[1] Other studies substantiate these figures.

A comparison of age-adjusted homicide rates indicates that the rates are lowest in New England (1.5 per 100,000), the West North Central states (2.9), and the Middle Atlantic states (3.2). (See Appendix Table 43.) Rates in the South are almost twice the rate of the United States as a whole; although the higher rates are sometimes attributed to the large proportion of Negro inhabitants, it should be noted that the rates for whites in the South are also much higher than for whites in the North. Highest rates among both white and nonwhite males per 100,000 population are in the East South Central (7.7 for whites, 50.9 for nonwhites) and West South Central (6.9 for whites, 51.7 for nonwhites) states; highest white and nonwhite female rates are in the Mountain (2.4 for whites, 12.1 for nonwhites) and South Atlantic (2.1 for whites, and 13.0 for nonwhites) states. (See Appendix Table 43.)

Foreign-born whites have somewhat higher rates than native-born whites in the East North Central area and lower rates in the South Atlantic and East South Central divisions (see Appendix Table 42). Rates for the foreign-born are highest in the West South Central states, where they exceed those of the native-born by a considerable amount.

Of the 50 states and the District of Columbia, the highest age-adjusted homicide rates are in Georgia (12.1 per 100,000), followed by Alabama (11.8), Mississippi (11.3), and the District of Columbia (11.2). The lowest rates are in Vermont, New Hampshire, Massachusetts, and Iowa: all are less than 1.4 (see Appendix Table 43).

Total homicide rates are similar for metropolitan and nonmetropolitan counties, but differences occur in some age groups. For instance, the metropolitan rate per 100,000 population for infants is almost twice the nonmetropolitan rate (4.3 and 2.6, respectively). When metropolitan counties with and without a central city are considered, differences are more pronounced: rates are consistently higher in those with a central city even when age, color, and sex are considered (see Appendix Table 40). Gangsterism and organized criminal behavior, sectional variations and location within a city, and the influence of cultural areas like slums have all been cited as explanations of the greater incidence of homicide in urban areas.

There is no significant evidence to uphold theories that the effect of season, temperature, barometric pressure, and humidity on the emotional state of the individual contribute to homicide.[2] Data in Appendix Table 44 indicate that rates are slightly higher in the summer and the month of December than at other times, and that they are lowest in the spring.

The homicide death rate today is about the same as it was in 1907. It increased rather consistently from 1900 (1.2 per 100,000) until about 1933 (9.8), decreased to about 1944 (5.0), and then increased somewhat until 1946 (6.4). Then it declined to a low of 4.5 in 1955, remaining substantially steady thereafter except for an increase to 4.9 in 1963. The pattern by color and sex has remained the same.[3] Comparisons of assault and criminal homicide statistics from *Uniform Crime Reports* for 1963 suggest that a potential victim is now likely to remain an assault statistic instead of becoming a homicide statistic; this might be attributable to improvements in fields of communications, medical technology, and police service.[4]

Information is lacking from which to determine whether a certain method of homicide is used by an offender in preference to another because his cultural background predisposes him to such a choice, because of accessibility of the weapon, or for some other reason. Nevertheless, available statistics indicate that firearms were the predominant method of killing during the early part of the century and that they still are.

Summary of the literature

Some studies have compared certain characteristics such as age, color, and sex of victims of criminal homicide with those of their killers. These studies fall into three general categories: those designed to develop insight into behavioral patterns affecting homicide; those that expose and correct common misconceptions; and those that suggest blueprints for the future formulation and evaluation of related hypotheses.

As an example of the results of such studies, there is a common misconception that homicide is largely interracial; but statistics from the Federal Bureau of Investigation and from individual studies show that it is more often intraracial and, further, that the victim is usually known personally to the offender and is frequently a member of the same family. It should perhaps be noted here again that these generalizations are based on homicides in which the killer has been identified.

In a study of 673 homicide victims and their 821 "offenders" in

North Carolina, Harold Garfinkel found that 90 percent of the cases were intraracial. Of the 821 offenders, almost 71 percent were Negroes whose victims were Negro; 20 percent were whites with white victims. Negro offenders whose victims were white were involved in 6 percent of the cases, and white offenders against Negroes in 3 percent. Two-thirds of all the cases studied involved males of the same race. The victims of female slayers were usually males, almost always members of the same race.[5] Bensing and Schroeder's study of 662 homicides in Cleveland[6] and Marvin Wolfgang's study of 588 cases in Philadelphia[7] have unearthed substantially the same statistics.

According to FBI data, about 60 percent of murder victims are within the age group 20-45: there are almost equal numbers in each 5-year grouping. Of persons arrested for murder, the greatest numbers are in the age group 20-24, followed by the 25-29 group with decreasing numbers thereafter.[8] Wolfgang found that the 20-24 group had the highest number of offenders and the 25-34 group the most victims; further, female offenders were older than female victims.[9] In Bensing and Schroeder's study, persons accused of felonious homicide were relatively young: 72 percent were aged 21-45 and 87 percent 16-50. The highest percentages were in the 26-30 (21 percent) and the 31-35 (19 percent) groups and the lowest were in the group 76 and over (0.2 percent). Of the decedents, 81 percent were 15-45.[10]

Of the 500 identified victim-offender relationships in Wolfgang's homicide study, most (over half) were in a primary group: that is, they were close friends or relatives. Five police-recorded motives— vaguely defined altercation, domestic quarrel, jealousy, argument over money, and robbery—were involved in eight out of ten cases of criminal homicide and were "more personalized when directed against or by women."[11]

On a national scale, the 1963 *Uniform Crime Reports* estimates a total of 8,500 offenses of murder and nonnegligent manslaughter for that year. This total was distributed according to victim-offender relationships or the motives involved, and the approximate distribution follows: those that occurred within the family unit, 31 percent; felony murders, 12 percent; altercations outside the family but usually among acquaintances, 51 percent; those in which no specific motive was determined at the time of reporting, 5 percent.

Of the offenses occurring within the family unit, approximately 53 percent were spouse killings; 17 percent involved the killing of children by parents; 6 percent were parricide cases; and 24 percent were killings among other relatives. Of the slayings outside the family unit that were identified a large proportion involved lovers' quarrels and drinking situations.[12]

A review of selected literature indicates that murderers usually have a crime record, although they may have never been institutionalized. A study by John Gillin of the Wisconsin "lifer" shows that in two out of three cases the murderer had never had previous institutional experience but that there was one chance in four that he had been arrested more than twice.[13]

A relatively high proportion of the offenders *and* victims studied by Wolfgang had police records—nearly two-thirds of the offenders and one-half of the victims. A greater proportion of Negro victims (male and female) had previous arrest records than white offenders of both sexes. When an offender had a police record it was more likely to be against person than property, and more likely than not it was a serious assault offense.[14]

In their study, Bensing and Schroeder found a high positive correlation between homicide and an index of social maladjustment—juvenile delinquency, child neglect and dependency, private-agency child placing, and illegitimate birth rate.[15]

Although a number of studies have sought to discern a relation between degree of education or intelligence and homicide, the evidence at hand is not conclusive. Where a relation appears to exist, it may be that there are differences in rates of conviction between social classes or races that affect the figures. This should be kept in mind when considering Bensing's and Schroeder's finding that areas with the highest homicide rates also have the largest proportions of persons who did not reach high school,[16] and Berg's and Fox's finding that convicted murderers in the State Prison of Southern Michigan scored significantly lower on tests of school achievement and intelligence than a random sample of the total prison population.[17] The same possibility should be applied to Gillin's finding that the educational level of 92 convicted murderers at Waupun, Wisconsin, was about the same as that of all prisoners in the United States committed for "grave homicide" but lower than that of males committed for all crimes.[18]

Studies indicate that many unfavorable elements usually exist in the home life of murderers: Gillin's study (which concentrates on 92 murderers in Wisconsin) indicates that in seven out of ten cases the convicted murderer had such a background. For example, the mother had worked outside the home during the subject's boyhood in almost twice as many cases as the average for all mothers in the United States. The subject had often had to assume early economic responsibility for family support; in seven out of ten cases he was 14 years of age when he began, and in over nine out of ten cases he contributed to family earnings before he was 21. Furthermore, there was one chance in three that his family had had a history of intemperance and at least one chance in five of insanity, epilepsy, or mental defect in his ancestry.

In a comparison of these murderers with their brothers, Gillin found that the murderers left school earlier, had full-time jobs before the age of 14 in significantly greater numbers, married women with more education than they themselves had had in significantly greater numbers, lived less harmoniously with their wives, and remained on their jobs for shorter periods of time than did their brothers.[19] While such a study is too limited to be conclusive, it does indicate areas deserving of greater exploration—especially in comparison with the noninstitutionalized population.

Studies of the density of population in areas where offenders reside, the socioeconomic status of the areas, conditions of housing, and other elements yield interesting results. In their study Bensing and Schroeder found that homicides were most prevalent in areas populated by Negroes and least prevalent in areas populated predominantly by native-born whites. For the most part, the Negroes lived in areas of greatest social need, poorest health, and greatest amount of substandard housing. The authors found that, in both Cleveland and Cuyahoga County (Ohio) as a whole, areas where homicides occurred most frequently were those most densely populated; sparsely populated areas had quite low homicide rates. High rates and overcrowded housing were closely correlated, and substandard housing related significantly to the problem. The study indicates that the lower the socioeconomic status of an area, the higher its homicide rate is.[20]

Cultural patterns, degree of external restraint (see definition of Henry and Short, below), tradition of violence, and the like, are not easily quantifiable; therefore their role in the perpetuation of the crime among groups where homicide rates are unusually high is difficult to evaluate. Nevertheless, many researchers believe that homicide is an outgrowth of a combination of determinants such as these, which subjectively define behavior acceptable to one's group.

H. C. Brearley hypothesizes that homicide rates are probably increased by the strength of certain cultural patterns that either "predispose or incite to deeds of violence," and that "these cultural patterns are often an indication of the presence of a social group with mores or social standards antagonistic to the rules and customs of a larger society."[21]

Elaborating on this theme, Wolfgang suggests that "a sub-culture of violence exists among a certain portion of the lower socio-economic group—especially comprised of males and Negroes. The social controls of the larger community are weakened in this sub-cultural milieu; and aggression, manifested in terms of homicidal assaults, is heightened."[22] These facts might account, in part at least, for differences found by researchers in homicide rates of various socioeconomic areas.

In his study of Negro and white crime rates in socioeconomically equated areas, Earl Moses points out that such external factors as housing and urban blight do not include subjective aspects like cultural meanings that are basic to the behavior patterns characteristic of a given group. His contention is that Negroes in these areas "due to a low socio-economic status accentuated by racial prescriptions . . . even as elsewhere, do not have a freedom of wholesome expression comparable to that of a similarly situated white group."[23]

According to Henry and Short, the degree of external restraint, or "the degree to which behavior is required to conform to the demands and expectations of others in the external world," distinguishes individuals who choose to commit homicide from those whose choice is suicide. They postulate that the more an individual has been externally restrained, the more he regards others as legitimate targets for aggression in response to his own frustration; consequently, it is more likely that he will commit homicide than suicide.[24]

Martin Gold has conducted a study based on the rationale that the kind of disciplinary measures taken against a child is both an index to and a factor in his shaping of values concerning expression of aggression. Furthermore, the study indicates that physical punishment in childhood leads to outward expressions (homicide), whereas psychological punishment turns aggression inward (suicide). In this frame of reference, Gold has constructed a "suicide-murder ratio"—an indication of preference for suicide over homicide—obtained by dividing the annual suicide rate for whites and nonwhites by the sum of that rate and the comparable homicide rate, using vital statistics for the years 1930-1940. He concludes that in every year from 1930 to 1940 whites, females, army officers, and urbanites clearly chose suicide over homicide more often than did nonwhites, males, enlisted men, and rural dwellers.[25]

8 / DISCUSSION

The foregoing chapters have described the problem of accidental injuries in the United States and elsewhere and have illustrated their toll in terms of death, hospitalization, and impairment; some of the problems of homicide have also been discussed. There are, undoubtedly, many social and psychological factors common to homicide and accidents, but the discussion in this chapter will be limited to the need for program development and research in the area of accidental injury.

In the discussion of particular types of accidents above, some known facts and some hypotheses that have been advanced regarding accident causation have been mentioned. The multiplicity of factors affecting causation should not discourage health departments and others from attempting to carry out programs of prevention. The great number of links in the chain of causation may make location of a weak link easier rather than more difficult.

Much is known about accident causation that can be translated into immediate programs of prevention. The facts are described in a recent book entitled *Accident Prevention*,[1] published for the American Public Health Association in cooperation with the Public Health Service; they are also treated in various publications of the Division of Accident Prevention, the National Safety Council, insurance companies, and other organizations. Some preventive measures have been developed for types of accidents for which cause and effect relations have been identified. Other measures are constantly being proposed in the hope of providing some degree of control, even though the underlying causes and interrelations of the accident types involved are not known. Nevertheless, much is still unknown regarding causation, and it is obvious that substantial research is necessary to produce the information needed by health departments and others for the implementation of prevention programs.

New methods and specific accident-prevention measures must be developed not only in the field of motor-vehicle accidents but for all other types of accidents as well. These must be based on adequate factual information provided by a vigorous program of accident-prevention research. It is clear that health agencies, concerned as they are with the health and well-being of man, should play a large role in accepting the responsibility of providing research and developing programs; and it seems reasonable to hope that they will do so. The orderly flow of information from research to program is extremely important, and the intermediate testing of prevention measures before their final incorporation into definitive programs is a task with which health departments are familiar.

The question of motivation is as acute in the field of accident prevention as in other fields of public health; in fact, the "prosaicness" of most accidents and the degree of active cooperation needed by the public may make the challenge here even more acute, and health educators and other behavioral scientists must rise to it. Developing a program to control accidental injury is a difficult job, requiring more tenacity and more hard work than many of the traditional health programs. Progress may be slow, but health departments and others cannot afford to wait until all the needed information is available—there will in fact never be such a time, as new hazards will arise while the old ones are being overcome. It is important to make use of whatever information is now available. The particular skills of health departments in community organization and education have already been demonstrated in the execution of many successful accident-prevention programs through the years.

An effective program of control involves not only prevention of the accident, but prevention of an injury or lessening of severity of an injury. In general, the reduction of disability, prolonged care, and impairment can be accomplished by use of safety equipment, adjustment of the environment or agent so that in an accident injury will be kept to a minimum, provision of immediate and adequate emergency medical service including first aid following an accident, and provision of adequate, definitive medical care thereafter to lessen the effects of injury. Both extensive research and the particular skills of the health educator are needed no less in such areas of secondary prevention than they are in the primary prevention of the accident. Of course, physical and vocational rehabilitation are also involved; the need for research in this area is discussed by William Haddon and others in their book *Accident Research.*[2]

Obvious examples of secondary prevention of industrial accidents include the use of helmets, safety shoes, safety belts, and so on, which have the purpose of preventing or ameliorating injury. In the field of motor-vehicle accident prevention, increasing emphasis is being put on design of the auto to lessen its effect after an accident. Knowledge gained from studying force of impact of the human body against the car on the inside or against an object outside after ejection has led to suggestions regarding locks and other methods of keeping doors closed to prevent ejection and to the use of seat belts, padding on dashboards, devices to reduce ejection and diminish the force of impact with objects inside the car. Study of the effectiveness of collapsible steering wheels, shatter-proof windshield glass, and other devices aims at reduction of the seriousness of injury. The obvious problem of head injuries to motorcyclists has led to strong recommendations that helmets be used.

The provision of first aid and emergency medical service is, of course, of extreme importance, not only for persons accidentally injured but also in other medical emergencies. The Public Health Service maintains as part of its mission an Emergency Medical Services Program that conducts studies, demonstrations, and surveys to assist communities in the development of coordinated systems to assure persons injured of prompt and proper aid at the scene of injury or emergency, safe and expeditious transportation, and proper hospital emergency medical care. In cooperation with medical societies, trauma committees, and health departments, studies are carried out in states and communities with improvement of the quality of available emergency medical service their objective. Training programs for ambulance personnel and others who can provide immediate care are conducted or supported.

The immediate goal of research into accident causation is to identify the factors associable with accidental injuries in the hope that their elimination or modification will reduce frequency and severity of injury. Thus human lives can be saved; and decreased impairment or disability and increased productivity following an accident can result. A great deal of data has been tabulated on fatalities and, somewhat more recently, injuries by characteristics of persons injured and by geographic distribution. Although such tabulations identify problem areas and the urgency of control measures, they rarely provide solutions or identify causal relations.

Because of the relatively recent recognition of accidents and other environmental hazards as major problems in public health today, there has been some lag in the recognition that accidents are, unfortunately, part of our way of life and of our cultural heritage. In spite of the extent of the accidental death and injury problem in the United States, causation research has been inadequate—to a large extent because of lack of interest in the accident problem on the part of researchers, lack of trained researchers and training facilities, and lack of specific hypotheses to be tested. Much existent research was conducted by physicians and others who are in constant contact with the results of accidental injury and who feel obligated to do something about it, even though they are often equipped with little else but enthusiasm and dedication. The extension of epidemiologic studies is needed to identify factors (especially host factors) that can be associated with different types of accidents, and to develop hypotheses and relationships that can be tested by the most stringent statistical methods possible and by controlled experimentation in the community and in research facilities.

One factor that has received much attention in literature and discussion—and a very important one in research toward accident prevention—is the classification of accidents and the problem of selecting events to be aggregated for analytical purposes. Obviously, the less homogeneous the family of accidents the more difficult it is to identify common causes; therefore classification into somewhat homogeneous categories is necessary for profitable research. There is no one grouping of accidents for all purposes, and it is essential to realize that the appropriateness of whatever classification is used depends upon the hypotheses, associations, or relationships being sought out or tested.

A very important item to be considered in this regard is the severity of the injury. As mentioned earlier, some types of accidents under some circumstances cause death and serious injury, but the same accident under other circumstances and to other people may cause minor injuries; it is important for the researcher to decide in advance whether he is looking for the characteristics and circumstances of the one kind of accident or of the other. The literature available has been dominated by theories of accident proneness, accident susceptibility, and the like; such theories imply that there is a continuum of accidental injuries with results from "ouch" to death and that the study of one produces information regarding the others. There is no evidence that this is so.

It is important, as mentioned earlier, that host and other factors be considered in selecting types of accidents for research. There is much evidence that falls to children and falls to elderly people have very little in common, so that research carried out on one age group may have no application to another; the same is true of motor-vehicle pedestrian accidents. Again, there may be very little in common between accidents to young people involving running off the roadway at 2 o'clock in the morning and collisions between two vehicles carrying middle-aged people in the afternoon. It is possible that lack of discrimination of types of accidents—including consideration of the persons to whom they happen and the circumstances under which they happen—may be responsible for misleading information and false hypotheses in the field of accident research.

In our modern, complex society accidents will always be a problem; as technology and customs change new accident problems will arise, and research programs will have to keep pace with corresponding changes in accident patterns. The following quotation, taken from *The Tribune* of Gallipolis, Ohio, illustrates the truth of this statement: "The number of serious . . . accidents is appalling. Fractured skulls, broken limbs, mutilated faces and ears torn off and spines crippled, are the daily record. And almost without exception every accident is the result of fast and reckless . . . ." The year was 1897; the agent was the bicycle.

Here, then, is a challenge to health workers to address themselves to an ever-changing problem. Challenge is not new to public health, nor, in fact, is change: the translation of efforts from the control of communicable diseases to the control of chronic diseases to the control of health hazards associated with environment is part of our heritage. Myron Wegman, Dean of the Michigan School of Public Health, quotes from *Travels with Charley,* by John Steinbeck, in a recent article called "The Changing Nature of Public Health": " 'It is the nature of men . . . to protest against change. . . . The sad ones are those who waste their energy in trying to hold it back, for they can only feel bitterness in loss and no joy in gain.' " Dr. Wegman then adds, "I have confidence that public health people will indeed feel the joy, for they, in the very nature of things, have change as their goal."[3]

REFERENCES

Chapter 1

1. Abel Wolman, "Public Health in Transition: Challenge and–Response?" *American Journal of Public Health,* 53:799-800 (May 1963).

2. John E. Gordon, "Changing Accents in Community Disease," *American Journal of Public Health,* 53:141-147 (February 1963).

3. Saad M. Gadalla, "Selected Environmental Factors Associated With Farm and Farm Home Accidents in Missouri" (Rural Health Series Publication 16, Research Bulletin 790; University of Missouri, January 1962).

4. Bruce D. Waxman, Robert J. Keehn, and Alexander J. Tutles, "Family Injury Survey: Preliminary Report, Prospective Study of Relationship between Occurrence of Accidents and Measurable Human Characteristics," *Connecticut Health Bulletin,* 72 (June 1958).

5. *Accident Facts* (Chicago: National Safety Council, 1966), p. 2.

6. *Impairments Due to Injury: July 1959-June 1961.* National Center for Health Statistics: Vital and Health Statistics. PHS Pub. No. 1000-Series 10-No. 6. (Washington, D. C.: Public Health Service, January 1964).

7. Commission on Military Accidents, Director's Summary Report to the Armed Forces Epidemiological Board, 1963-1964.

8. *Medical Statistics: U.S. Navy* (Statistical Report of the Surgeon General, U.S. Navy). *Annual Report of the U.S.A.F. Medical Service* (Office of the Surgeon General, U.S. Air Force). *Health of the Army* (Office of the Surgeon General, Department of the Army).

9. Joseph E. Barmack and Donald E. Payne, "The Lackland Accident Countermeasure Experiment," *Highway Research Board Proceedings,* 40:513-522 (1961).

10. *Epidemiological and Vital Statistics Report* (Geneva: World Health Organization, 1965), 18:117-124.

11. Mortimer Spiegelman, "Mortality Trends for Causes of Death in Countries of Low Mortality," *Demography,* 2:115-125 (1965).

Chapter 2

1. Brian MacMahon, Thomas F. Pugh, and Johannes Ipsen, *Epidemiologic Methods* (Boston: Little, Brown and Company, 1960), p. 3.

2. John E. Gordon, "The Epidemiology of Accidents," *American Journal of Public Health,* 39:504-515 (April 1949).

3. William Haddon, Jr., Edward A. Suchman, and David Klein, *Accident Research: Methods and Approaches* (New York: Harper and Row, 1964), p. 378.

Chapter 3

1. *Planned Pedestrian Program* (Washington, D. C.: The American Automobile Association Foundation for Traffic Safety, 1958), pp. 18-20.

2. *Trends in Indian Health and Health Services* (Washington, D. C.: Public Health Service, 1965).

3. Mindel C. Sheps, "Marriage and Mortality," *American Journal of Public Health,* 51:547-555 (April 1961).

4. Joseph Berkson, "Mortality and Marital Status—Reflections on the Derivation of Etiology from Statistics," *American Journal of Public Health,* 52:1318-1329 (August 1962).

5. Aluert P. Iskrant, "Accident Mortality Data as Epidemiologic Indicators," *American Journal of Public Health,* 50:161-172 (February 1960).

6. Abel Wolman, "Public Health in Transition: Challenge and—Response?" *American Journal of Public Health,* 53:799-800 (May 1963).

7. Lillian Guralnick, "Occupations of Men Dying from Accidents in the United States, 1950," *Public Health Reports,* 76:817-823 (September 1961).

8. William S. Langford, Rodman Gilder, Jr., Virginia N. Wilking, Minnie Marder Genn, and Helen H. Sherrill, "Pilot Study of Childhood Accidents: Preliminary Report," *Pediatrics,* 11:405-415 (April 1953).

9. E. Maurice Backett and A. M. Johnston. "Social Patterns of Road Accidents to Children—Some Characteristics of Vulnerable Families," *British Medical Journal* (February 14, 1959), pp. 409-413.

10. Morris S. Schulzinger, "The Pre-Accident Patient: Diagnosis and Treatment," *Industrial Medicine and Surgery,* 25:451-458 (October 1956).

11. Edward A. Suchman, "Cultural and Social Factors in Accident Occurrence and Control," *Journal of Occupational Medicine,* 7:487-492 (October 1965).

12. Ross A. McFarland and Roland C. Moore, *Youth and the Automobile* (New York: Association for the Aid of Crippled Children, 1960), pp. 1-16.

13. H. Laurence Ross, "Traffic Law Violation: A Folk Crime," *Social Problems,* 8:231-241 (Winter 1961).

14. Ross A. McFarland, Roland C. Moore, and A. Bertrand Warren, *Human Variables in Motor Vehicle Accidents: A Review of the Literature* (Boston: Harvard School of Public Health, 1955), p. 43.

15. Jerome J. Beamish and James L. Malfetti, "A Psychological Comparison of Violator and Non-Violator Automobile Drivers in the 16 to 19 Year Age Group," *Traffic Safety Research Review* (March 1962), pp. 12-15.

16. John J. Conger, Herbert S. Gaskill, Donald D. Glad, Linda Hassel, Robert V. Rainey, William L. Sawrey, and Eugene S. Turrell, "Psychological and Psychophysiological Factors in Motor Vehicle Accidents," *The Journal of the American Medical Association,* 169:1581-1587 (April 4, 1959).

17. W. A. Tillmann and G. E. Hobbs, "The Accident-Prone Automobile Driver," *The American Journal of Psychiatry,* 106:321-331 (November 1949).

18. Vita Krall, "Personality Characteristics of Accident Repeating Children," *The Journal of Abnormal and Social Psychology,* 48:99-107 (January 1953).

19. Lawrence L. LeShan, "Dynamics in Accident-Prone Behavior," *Psychiatry,* 15:73-80 (1952).

20. Flanders Dunbar, "The Relationship Between Anxiety States and Organic Disease," *Clinics,* 1:879-908 (December 1942).

21. Irwin M. Marcus, Wilma Wilson, Irvin Kraft, Delmar Swander, Fred Southerland, and Edith Schulhofer, "An Interdisciplinary Approach to Accident Patterns in Children," *Monographs of the Society for Research in Child Development,* 25:1-79 (1960).

22. Fletcher D. Woodward, Horace E. Campbell, Jacob Kulowski, Harold M. Brandaleone, John R. Rodger, Seward E. Miller, Ross A. McFarland, James L. Goddard, and Howard N. Schulz, "Medical Guide for Physicians in Determining Fitness to Drive a Motor Vehicle," *The Journal of the American Medical Association,* 169:1195-1207 (March 14, 1959).

23. Selwyn D. Collins, "Relation of Chronic Disease and Socioeconomic Status to Accident Liability," *Public Health Monograph No. 14* (Washington, D. C.: U. S. Department of Health, Education and Welfare, Public Health Service, March 1953), pp. 43-65.

24. Katharina Dalton, "Menstruation and Accidents," *Accident Research: Methods and Approaches* (New York: Harper and Row, 1964), pp. 201-205.

25. Albert P. Iskrant, "Relationship Between Medical Conditions and Accidental Injuries" (address to the Governor's Traffic Safety Conference, Sacramento, California, 1959).

26. Bonita J. Peterson and Charles S. Petty, "Sudden Natural Death Among Automobile Drivers," *Journal of Forensic Sciences,* 7:274-285 (July 1962).

27. S. R. Gerber, Paul V. Joliet, and John R. Feegel, "Single Motor Vehicle Accidents in Cuyahoga County (Ohio): 1958-1963," *Journal of Forensic Sciences,* 11:144-151 (April 1966).

28. Julian A. Waller, "Chronic Medical Conditions and Traffic Safety—Review of the California Experience," *The New England Journal of Medicine,* 273: 1413-1420 (December 23, 1965).

29. Richard G. Domey and James E. Duckworth, "Comparative Study of Highway Accidents Among 625 Physically Impaired Licensees Matched with 625 Nonimpaired Licensees," unpublished manuscript, Harvard School of Public Health, Boston, August 1, 1963.

30. Woodward *et al.,* "Medical Guide for Physicians," 1195-1207.

31. Leonard Colebrook and Vera Colebrook, "The Prevention of Burns and Scalds—Review of 1000 Cases," *The Lancet* (July 30, 1949), pp. 181-188.

32. "Accidental Falls trom Windows," *Statistical Bulletin* of the Metropolitan Life Insurance Company, 33:6-7 (February 1952).

33. J. H. Sheldon, "On the Natural History of Falls in Old Age," *British Medical Journal* (December 10, 1960), pp. 1685-1690.

34. I. Jay Brightman, Isabel McCaffrey, and Leonard P. Cook, "Mortality Statistics as a Direction Finder in Home Accident Prevention," *American Journal of Public Health,* 42:840-848 (July 1952).

Chapter 4

1. *Summary and Analysis of Accidents on Railroads in the United States Subject to the Interstate Commerce Act* (Interstate Commerce Commission, Bureau of Railroad Safety and Service; Accident Bulletin No. 133, 1964).

2. *Accident Facts* (Chicago: National Safety Council, 1966), p. 41.

3. William Haddon, Jr., Preston Valien, James R. McCarroll, and Charles J. Umberger, "A Controlled Investigation of the Characteristics of Adult Pedestrians Fatally Injured by Motor Vehicles in Manhattan," *Journal of Chronic Diseases,* 14:655-678 (December 1961).

4. J. Stannard Baker, "Case Studies of Traffic Accidents," *Traffic Safety Research Review,* 5:14-17 (December 1961).

5. Haddon *et al.,* "Adult Pedestrians Fatally Injured." James R. McCarroll and William Haddon, Jr., "A Controlled Study of Fatal Automobile Accidents in New York City," *Journal of Chronic Diseases,* 15:811-826 (August 1962).

6. John J. Conger, "Research Trends in Traffic Safety," *Traffic Safety Research Review,* 5:30-32 (June 1961).

7. Frederick L. McGuire, "A Psychological Comparison of Accident-Violation Free and Accident-Incurring Automobile Drivers" (Naval Medical Field Research Laboratory, Camp LeJeune, North Carolina; 6:1-26, February 1955).

8. Ross A. McFarland, Roland C. Moore, and A. Bertrand Warren, *Human Variables in Motor Vehicle Accidents: A Review of the Literature* (Boston: Harvard School of Public Health, 1955).

9. Leon G. Goldstein, *Research on Human Variables in Safe Motor Vehicle Operation: A Correlational Summary of Predictor Variables and Criterion Measures* (Washington, D. C.: George Washington University, 1961).

10. Walter A. Merriam and Jules V. Quint, "Factors Bearing on the Underwriting of Accident Risks" (address to the Annual Meeting of the Home Office Life Underwriters Association, Toronto, Ontario, Canada, May 1962).

11. *Automotive Crash Injury Research* (Buffalo: Cornell Aeronautical Laboratory, Cornell University, March 1, 1961).

12. *Nosology Guidelines.* National Center for Health Statistics: Supplement to the Cause-of-Death Coding Manual (Washington, D. C.: Public Health Service, August 1960), p. 2.

13. Albert P. Iskrant, William C. James, and Jewel G. Wyman, "An Epidemiologic Investigation of 5,000 Non-Motor Vehicle Injuries" (address to the Ninety-First Annual Meeting of the American Public Health Association, Kansas City, Missouri, November 12, 1963).

14. "Bicycle Accident Statistics," *Safety Education,* 38:6-12 (January 1959).

15. "Report of the Committee on Aviation: Aviation Statistics," *Society of Actuaries Transactions: 1964 Reports of Mortality and Morbidity Statistics* (June 1965).

16. Charles R. Harper and William R. Albers, "Alcohol and General Aviation Accidents," *Aerospace Medicine,* 35:462-464 (May 1964).

17. Norman Heaton, "Parachuting Statistics—Part I: Fatalities," *Parachutist* (February 1966), pp. 2, 17-19.

18. Bramwell W. Gabrielson, *Facts on Drowning Accidents* (Athens, Georgia: University of Georgia, 1956), p. 51.

19. Warren W. Morse, "Epidemiological Notes: Accidental Drownings at Home," *Public Health Reports,* 76:452 (May 1961).

20. "Report of California Drownings—1963," *California's Health,* 22:22 (August 1, 1964).

21. "Accidental Drownings Occurring in Florida" (Florida State Board of Health, Monthly Statistical Report, April 23, 1964).

22. "Many Drownings Among Young Children," *Statistical Bulletin* of the Metropolitan Life Insurance Company, 34:9-10 (July 1953).

23. Gabrielson, *Facts on Drowning Accidents,* p. 55.

24. *Recreational Boating in the United States: A Report on Accidents, Numbering and Related Activities, CG-357* (Washington, D. C.: U.S. Coast Guard, May 1, 1965), pp. 15-17.

25. G. Dekle Taylor, Everett H. Williams, Jr., and G. Lindsey Chappell, "Skin and Scuba Diving Fatalities," *The Journal of the Florida Medical Association,* 49:808-810 (April 1963).

26. Julian A. Waller, Paul Caplan, and A. E. Lowe, *Skin and Scuba Diving As a Health Problem* (Berkeley: State of California Department of Public Health, January 2, 1964), pp. 1-32.

27. Myron K. Denney and Raymond C. Read, "Scuba-Diving Deaths in Michigan," *The Journal of the American Medical Association,* 192:120-122 (April 19, 1965).

28. Gabrielson, *Facts on Drowning Accidents,* p. 58.

29. Wayne DeWitte Cross, "Accidental Drownings in Iowa, 1950-1963, With Case Studies Involving Those Under 10 Years of Age," unpublished dissertation, Iowa State University, Ames, Iowa, 1964.

30. Gabrielson, *Facts on Drowning Accidents,* p. 49.

31. Howard M. Cann, Albert P. Iskrant, and Dorothy S. Neyman, "Epidemiologic Aspects of Poisoning Accidents," *American Journal of Public Health,* 50: 1914-1924 (December 1960).

32. Albert P. Iskrant, "Accident Mortality Data as Epidemiologic Indicators," *American Journal of Public Health,* 50:161-172 (February 1960).

33. Albert P. Iskrant, "The Etiology of Fractured Hips in Females" (address to the Ninety-Fourth Annual Meeting of the American Public Health Association, San Francisco, California, November 3, 1966).

34. Trevor H. Howell, "Old Folk Who Fall," *The Practitioner,* 175:56-58 (July 1955).

35. C. A. Boucher, "Falls in the Home," *The Medical Officer,* 102:194-195 (October 16, 1959).

36. Michael Gyepes, Harry Z. Mellins, and Isadore Katz, "The Low Incidence of Fracture of the Hip in the Negro," *The Journal of the American Medical Association,* 181:133-134 (September 22, 1962).

37. Joseph A. Miller and Merle L. Esmay, "Stairway Falls," *Home Safety Review,* 16:23-25 (Winter 1958).

38. *Comparability of Mortality Statistics for the Sixth and Seventh Revisions:* United States, 1958. National Center for Health Statistics: Vital Statistics—Special Reports, Vol. 51, No. 4 (Washington, D. C.: Public Health Service, March 1965).

39. *Accident Facts,* p. 31.

40. Warren W. Morse, "Epidemiological Notes: Deaths from Electric Current," *Public Health Reports,* 75:962 (October 1960).

41. "Accidental Death From Electric Current," *Statistical Bulletin* of the Metropolitan Life Insurance Company, 36:8-10 (May 1955).

42. "Estimated U.S. Building Fire Losses by Causes, 1964," *Fire Journal,* 59:32 (September 1965).

43. John C. McLeish, Barbara J. Ashenden, and Leon Eisenberg, "A Clinical Investigation of Firesetting by Children," *Research Relating to Children* (Children's Bureau, Washington, D. C.; Bulletin 9), p. 32.

44. Julian A. Waller and Dean I. Manheimer, "Nonfatal Burns of Children in a Well-Defined Urban Population," *The Journal of Pediatrics,* 65:863-869 (December 1964).

45. Ethel J. Alpenfels and Arthur B. Hayes, III, "Cultural Factors Affecting Accidents Among Children," *Behavioral Approaches to Accident Research* (New York: New York Association for the Aid of Crippled Children, 1961), pp. 103-109.

46. *Firearm Fatalities* (Jefferson City: Missouri Department of Public Health and Welfare, 1961), pp. 1-17.

47. "How Fatal Accidents Occur in the Home," *Statistical Bulletin* of the Metropolitan Life Insurance Company, 40:6-8 (November-December 1959).

48. *Uniform Hunter Casualty Report* (Washington, D. C.: The National Rifle Association, 1963), pp. 1-34.

49. Henry M. Parrish, John C. Goldner, and Stanley L. Silberg, "Comparison Between Snakebites in Children and Adults," *Pediatrics,* 36:251-256 (August 1965).

50. *Accidental Death and Injury Statistics.* PHS Pub. No. 1111 (Washington, D. C.: Public Health Service, Division of Accident Prevention, October 1963), p. 41.

51. "Storms and Floods Take Fewer Lives," *Statistical Bulletin* of the Metropolitan Life Insurance Company, 45:8-10 (April 1964).

Chapter 5

1. *Accident Facts* (Chicago: National Safety Council, 1966), p. 23.

2. *Ibid.,* p. 3.

3. *Ibid.,* p. 23.

4. "American Standard Method of Compiling Industrial Injury Rates," *American Safety Standards* of the American Standards Association, Z16.1 (1945).

5. *Accident Facts,* p. 24.

6. *Ibid.,* p. 23.

7. *Ibid.,* p. 25.

8. "Competitive Sports and Their Hazards," *Statistical Bulletin* of the Metropolitan Life Insurance Company, 46:1-3 (September 1965).

9. William Haddon, Jr., Arthur E. Ellison, and Robert E. Carroll, "Skiing Injuries," *Public Health Reports,* 77:975-991 (November 1962).

10. A. Scott Earle, John R. Moritz, George B. Saviers, and James D. Ball, "Ski Injuries," *The Journal of the American Medical Association,* 180:285-288 (April 28, 1962).

11. B. G. Ferris, Jr., "Hazards to Health: Mountain-Climbing Accidents in the United States," *The New England Journal of Medicine,* 268:430-431 (February 21, 1963).

12. "Competitive Sports and Their Hazards," *Statistical Bulletin* of the Metropolitan Life Insurance Company, 46:1-3 (September 1965).

13. H. W. Mammen, "The Need for Employee Health Services in Hospitals," *Archives of Environmental Health,* 9:750-757 (December 1964).

Chapter 6

1. *Types of Injuries: July 1957-June 1961.* National Center for Health Statistics: Vital and Health Statistics. PHS Pub. No. 1000-Series 10-No. 8 (Washington, D.C.: Public Health Service, April 1964).

2. Dean I. Manheimer, Joanna Dewey, Glen D. Mellinger, and Leslie Corsa, Jr., "50,000 Child-Years of Accidental Injuries," *Public Health Reports,* 81:519-533 (June 1966).

3. Jaakko K. Kihlberg, *Head Injury in Automobile Accidents* (Buffalo: Cornell Aeronautical Laboratory Report No. VJ-1823-R17; Cornell University, November 1965).

4. *Impairments Due to Injury: July 1959-June 1961.* National Center for Health Statistics: Vital and Health Statistics. PHS Pub. No. 1000-Series 10-No. 6 (Washington, D.C.: Public Health Service, January 1964).

5. Berish Strauch, "Bicycle Spoke Injuries in Children," *The Journal of Trauma,* 6:61-64 (January 1966).

6. Unpublished tabulations, Illinois Department of Public Health, Springfield, Illinois.

7. *Types of Injuries: June 1957-June 1961.* National Center for Health Statistics: Vital and Health Statistics. PHS Pub. No. 1000-Series 10-No. 8 (Washington, D. C.: Public Health Service, April 1964).

Chapter 7

1. *Mortality by Occupation and Cause of Death among Men 20 to 64 Years of Age: United States, 1950.* National Center for Health Statistics: Vital Statistics—Special Reports, Vol. 53, No. 3 (Washington, D.C.: Public Health Service, September 1963).

2. Joseph Cohen, "The Geography of Crime," *The Annals of the American Academy of Political and Social Science,* 217:29-37 (September 1941).

3. *Death Rates by Age, Race, and Sex, United States, 1900-1953: Homicide.* National Center for Health Statistics: Vital Statistics—Special Reports, Vol. 43, No. 31 (Washington, D.C.: Public Health Service, August 23, 1956).

4. *Crime in the United States: Uniform Crime Reports* (Washington, D.C.: Federal Bureau of Investigation, 1963), p. 6.

5. Harold Garfinkel, "Research Note on Inter- and Intra-Racial Homicide," *Social Forces,* 27:369-381 (May 1949).

6. Robert S. Bensing and Oliver Schroeder, *Homicide in an Urban Community* (Springfield, Illinois: Charles C. Thomas, 1960), p. 100.

7. Marvin E. Wolfgang, *Patterns in Criminal Homicide* (Philadelphia: University of Pennsylvania Press, 1958), p. 325.

8. *Uniform Crime Reports,* p. 102.

9. Wolfgang, *Patterns in Criminal Homicide,* p. 320.

10. Bensing and Schroeder, *Homicide in an Urban Community,* p. 99.

11. Wolfgang, *Patterns in Criminal Homicide,* p. 324.

12. *Uniform Crime Reports,* pp. 6-7.

13. John L. Gillin, "Murder as a Sociological Phenomenon," *The Annals of the American Academy of Political and Social Science,* 284:20-25 (November 1952).

14. Wolfgang, *Patterns in Criminal Homicide,* pp. 323-324.

15. Bensing and Schroeder, *Homicide in an Urban Community,* p. 171.

16. *Ibid.,* p. 125.

17. Irwin A. Berg and Vernon Fox, "Factors in Homicides Committed by 200 Males," *The Journal of Social Psychology,* 26:109-119 (August 1947).

18. Gillin, "Murder as a Sociological Phenomenon," p. 21.

19. *Ibid.,* pp. 20-21.

20. Bensing and Schroeder, *Homicide in an Urban Community,* pp. 117-118 and 132-138.

21. H. C. Brearley, *Homicide in the United States* (Chapel Hill: University of North Carolina Press, 1932), p. 51.

22. Wolfgang, *Patterns in Criminal Homicide,* p. 330.

23. Earl R. Moses, "Differentials in Crime Rates Between Negroes and Whites, Based on Comparisons of Four Socio-Economically Equated Areas," *American Sociological Review,* 12:411-420 (August 1947).

24. Andrew F. Henry and James F. Short, Jr., *Suicide and Homicide* (Glencoe, Illinois: The Free Press, 1954), p. 120.

25. Martin Gold, "Suicide, Homicide and the Socialization of Aggression," *American Journal of Sociology,* 63:651-661 (May 1958).

Chapter 8

1. Maxwell N. Halsey, ed., *Accident Prevention: The Role of Physicians and Public Health Workers* (New York: McGraw-Hill, 1961).

2. William Haddon, Jr., Edward A. Suchman, and David Klein, *Accident Research: Methods and Approaches* (New York: Harper and Row, 1964), chap. ix, pp. 535-612.

3. Myron E. Wegman, "The Changing Nature of Public Health," *American Journal of Public Health,* 53:705-711 (May 1963).

STATISTICAL APPENDIX

Table 1 Death rates for all accidents, by age, color, and sex: United States, 1959-61
(E800-E962)

Age	Total			White			Nonwhite		
	Total	Male	Female	Total	Male	Female	Total	Male	Female
All ages	51.7	72.3	31.8	50.1	69.7	31.1	64.2	92.5	37.4
Under 1	91.4	100.9	81.6	75.3	84.1	66.2	183.2	199.2	167.3
1	41.2	45.5	36.7	36.4	40.4	32.3	69.0	75.7	62.2·
2	31.7	36.4	26.8	27.4	32.2	22.4	57.0	61.4	52.5
3	26.8	31.6	21.9	23.4	28.9	17.7	47.2	48.1	46.2
4	24.0	27.3	20.6	20.9	24.6	17.1	42.3	43.5	41.2
5 - 14	18.9	26.3	11.2	17.4	24.6	10.0	28.1	37.3	18.9
15 - 24	55.8	92.8	19.4	55.7	92.4	19.3	56.6	95.8	19.9
25 - 34	42.8	71.4	15.3	40.4	67.4	14.0	61.1	103.8	24.3
35 - 44	40.6	65.4	17.0	37.5	60.3	15.5	67.5	110.3	29.1
45 - 54	49.1	76.4	22.6	46.1	71.4	21.5	76.7	122.7	32.9
55 - 64	58.5	88.1	30.7	55.6	83.8	29.2	87.6	130.8	45.8
65 - 74	86.8	117.9	59.7	85.3	116.1	58.6	103.8	138.7	71.9
75 - 84	210.4	234.6	191.6	213.8	238.1	195.2	163.6	191.7	138.4
85 & over	625.3	588.9	648.6	650.7	612.8	674.5	321.5	335.9	310.4
Age-adjusted									
Total	49.4	73.3	26.4	47.3	70.2	25.1	65.5	98.6	34.9
Under 15	26.5	33.1	19.5	23.5	30.1	16.7	44.3	52.4	36.1
65 & over	39.8	166.4	116.8	140.6	167.0	118.0	127.7	160.1	98.3

Table 2   Death rates for all accidents, persons age 15 and over, by color, sex, and marital status:[a] United States, 1959-61 (E800-E962)

Age and sex	White					Nonwhite				
	Total	Single	Married	Widowed	Divorced	Total	Single	Married	Widowed	Divorced
Male	87.3	106.7	65.2	276.2	265.1	115.2	122.2	91.3	241.9	221.0
15 - 19	79.7	78.8	87.6	208.3*	141.8	79.3	77.2	96.4	330.7*	-
20 - 24	107.2	130.2	74.8	379.4	254.4	115.8	129.9	88.1	289.6*	188.6
25 - 29	73.5	103.7	60.6	330.3	233.5	109.2	149.4	85.3	309.5	215.5
30 - 34	61.9	93.2	52.8	207.9	218.2	99.9	150.5	80.1	210.9	160.9
35 - 39	58.4	93.8	48.8	192.7	234.2	108.4	180.9	85.1	195.8	203.0
40 - 44	62.5	107.2	51.6	168.1	249.2	114.2	211.0	87.3	261.4	230.2
45 - 49	67.9	114.5	54.8	164.7	274.4	119.8	220.4	93.5	245.6	191.6
50 - 54	74.5	124.8	59.3	171.0	265.1	127.3	188.3	98.3	241.7	248.9
55 - 59	79.1	126.8	62.6	163.4	255.8	119.2	142.7	91.3	224.7	231.3
60 - 64	88.9	144.4	69.5	162.1	268.3	143.8	208.2	103.1	243.0	308.6
65 - 69	106.7	194.7	79.8	183.6	288.9	133.5	215.5	91.2	221.3	279.6
70 - 74	134.1	239.7	96.8	203.1	331.6	147.6	252.3	106.0	195.9	252.9
75 - 79	207.4	331.3	150.4	280.8	414.5	170.5	249.0	126.3	213.6	215.0*
80 - 84	328.8	524.7	244.6	386.0	610.4	252.8	348.2	165.7	338.4	318.8*
85 & over	665.8	742.6	499.5	755.6	853.5	366.0	439.9	264.4	410.2	612.4*
Female	36.6	32.6	20.7	125.5	53.9	35.6	27.1	24.9	85.9	44.2
15 - 19	20.4	19.9	20.8	141.6*	75.7	17.7	17.1	18.0	82.0*	52.2*
20 - 24	18.0	23.2	14.3	101.2	60.2	22.7	25.9	18.8	65.8*	44.6*
25 - 29	14.3	20.2	12.1	65.0	55.4	23.0	35.4	19.3	50.9*	27.9
30 - 34	13.7	20.1	11.7	56.3	45.1	25.6	40.3	20.6	67.3	40.8
35 - 39	14.5	17.3	12.4	46.3	43.1	27.7	41.0	22.9	48.7	41.7
40 - 44	16.6	19.2	14.4	35.6	42.0	30.5	50.4	24.6	52.9	35.1
45 - 49	19.7	19.9	17.2	36.4	43.3	30.1	47.2	23.9	46.0	44.8
50 - 54	23.0	19.1	20.4	37.8	38.6	35.8	33.6	28.7	49.9	46.4
55 - 59	25.7	24.9	22.7	33.0	45.8	37.6	25.1	25.8	63.0	42.1
60 - 64	32.7	38.8	28.2	38.9	46.6	53.7	60.1	37.0	70.2	58.3*
65 - 69	44.9	50.3	39.2	50.2	53.8	60.9	67.9	44.4	71.5	81.7*
70 - 74	77.9	92.4	65.1	83.0	114.9	87.6	87.8	65.4	98.7	90.0*
75 - 79	143.7	180.4	119.7	147.0	185.4	119.4	106.1*	74.1	130.9	146.2*
80 - 84	306.8	363.7	268.7	303.8	400.5	180.1	196.7*	172.8	172.9	328.4*
85 & over	721.7	816.3	483.0	731.5	653.8	327.4	344.5*	141.6*	341.2	-

[a] Excludes "not stated."

Table 3   Death rates for all accidents, by age: United States,
each geographic division and state, 1959-61
(E800-E962)

Geographic area	All ages	Under 5	5-14	15-24	25-34	35-44	45-54	55-64	65-74	75-84	85 & over
United States	51.7	43.2	18.9	55.8	42.8	40.6	49.1	58.5	86.8	210.4	625.3
New England	44.2	32.7	14.5	40.7	25.4	25.2	33.3	45.2	85.6	238.8	702.7
Connecticut	36.4	26.1	11.4	38.3	24.7	23.1	30.1	39.9	71.6	206.3	530.0
Maine	52.6	48.8	22.9	58.7	42.6	37.0	54.2	48.3	72.0	183.9	439.0
Massachusetts	46.8	29.4	13.7	35.5	21.7	23.9	32.0	49.7	101.1	278.3	867.3
New Hampshire	45.5	43.4	17.8	68.3	37.4	28.0	28.8	30.8	63.6	175.6	494.4
Rhode Island	35.1	40.1	12.3	27.3	17.8	20.0	23.9	32.5	61.1	204.2	650.7
Vermont	56.5	45.6	22.9	60.3	36.4	39.0	51.7	61.4	79.1	211.0	668.1
Middle Atlantic	41.2	31.7	14.4	38.9	27.3	26.8	35.0	47.8	81.9	213.9	581.6
New Jersey	38.3	38.0	13.8	37.3	24.6	22.6	32.7	44.4	73.9	205.2	598.1
New York	40.4	28.7	13.8	37.0	27.3	26.6	34.0	46.7	80.9	210.0	578.7
Pennsylvania	44.0	32.5	15.6	42.4	28.7	29.4	37.8	51.6	87.4	223.5	577.8
East North Central	47.3	33.9	17.3	51.7	36.6	34.0	42.2	56.1	87.3	214.6	645.6
Illinois	42.3	31.7	16.1	46.0	34.6	32.6	39.8	52.2	74.8	167.6	400.1
Indiana	55.0	40.2	19.9	59.0	42.9	39.2	49.5	59.8	92.3	245.5	783.9
Michigan	47.0	37.0	17.6	51.7	36.1	34.6	42.4	57.2	93.9	225.8	751.1
Ohio	47.7	30.0	17.0	47.1	36.3	32.5	41.5	58.6	92.9	241.9	729.4
Wisconsin	50.8	35.5	17.1	67.6	36.1	34.4	42.1	54.7	89.9	210.5	694.4
West North Central	56.7	40.3	19.6	62.8	44.5	41.2	51.1	59.9	88.5	209.9	713.5
Iowa	56.0	39.2	20.0	62.6	40.8	40.1	50.4	54.8	80.9	202.2	729.6
Kansas	57.5	41.3	20.0	65.0	46.6	39.9	49.5	59.4	90.2	194.9	782.1
Minnesota	52.0	34.5	18.7	58.9	37.2	40.4	47.6	59.0	89.0	204.5	715.4
Missouri	58.5	45.5	18.3	58.1	44.7	41.0	52.5	60.9	90.3	225.6	713.7
Nebraska	56.4	38.5	17.2	65.5	45.6	39.1	49.3	60.6	88.4	212.2	659.4
North Dakota	60.4	41.9	27.0	65.9	55.5	54.4	58.6	67.7	106.6	214.4	570.1
South Dakota	66.9	43.3	25.5	95.7	76.1	49.0	64.2	73.3	87.0	203.1	593.0
South Atlantic	56.0	55.7	22.8	60.4	51.9	51.7	58.6	64.8	82.2	189.8	522.7
Delaware	44.4	28.3	16.3	53.0	40.1	34.1	45.3	54.2	35.1	167.6	603.7
District of Columbia	54.4	76.0	17.3	33.3	29.2	46.3	62.0	61.4	104.2	214.6	501.5
Florida	57.5	62.7	24.9	63.9	51.4	50.5	61.4	58.6	65.4	164.6	496.8
Georgia	59.3	61.0	25.0	63.6	58.8	56.4	63.9	70.5	83.9	189.0	504.7
Maryland	44.8	39.7	18.2	43.4	36.0	35.3	44.4	59.1	89.1	227.1	508.7
North Carolina	57.2	60.0	22.7	68.8	57.1	56.2	56.1	67.3	85.8	169.3	470.5
South Carolina	66.3	72.5	31.0	65.7	74.1	70.3	72.4	78.8	93.5	193.0	483.7
Virginia	51.7	43.9	18.4	54.4	46.0	47.1	54.5	62.1	90.5	217.4	607.0
West Virginia	59.8	44.0	22.0	66.1	52.6	59.2	64.4	71.2	87.6	198.0	597.5
East South Central	60.8	58.4	23.3	65.6	57.3	55.3	64.2	66.4	86.7	203.1	618.3
Alabama	62.6	61.6	25.2	66.0	64.3	59.3	67.5	75.1	89.8	190.0	553.8
Kentucky	61.8	48.0	19.1	69.8	52.8	50.7	64.0	65.3	93.5	234.6	805.2
Mississippi	69.1	80.6	29.7	69.8	69.2	69.1	72.2	69.8	91.3	210.2	497.6
Tennessee	53.4	48.5	20.7	59.0	48.4	48.2	57.0	58.1	74.9	179.0	563.8
West South Central	59.7	54.4	23.1	65.9	54.3	52.8	60.8	68.4	91.2	211.4	610.6
Arkansas	67.0	67.9	28.3	75.2	58.9	56.2	65.1	64.2	94.6	204.4	569.2
Louisiana	59.7	54.4	22.4	69.8	60.1	50.4	59.9	74.3	95.7	214.8	626.2
Oklahoma	67.6	54.7	24.0	70.7	54.4	53.9	71.7	75.0	99.5	214.2	714.9
Texas	56.5	52.2	22.2	61.7	51.8	52.7	57.3	65.4	86.2	211.2	576.1
Mountain	70.2	61.9	23.4	84.8	70.0	63.2	76.3	82.5	108.9	235.7	755.5
Arizona	69.0	75.1	20.2	83.7	72.8	67.6	81.8	80.8	101.6	185.2	562.1
Colorado	61.4	47.7	22.3	64.9	54.6	48.8	64.0	72.8	96.6	234.4	731.5
Idaho	74.7	69.8	29.9	89.0	65.7	61.8	80.1	83.1	119.3	227.3	782.6
Montana	81.5	59.8	27.8	114.4	85.2	72.5	81.0	88.5	113.2	232.2	809.6
Nevada	90.2	80.7	26.5	102.2	83.7	80.0	105.3	120.3	174.1	324.0	831.3
New Mexico	76.2	67.6	24.2	97.1	94.4	78.7	79.2	94.6	108.7	257.0	776.8
Utah	58.3	49.9	19.5	67.0	51.7	51.2	68.1	67.8	107.5	258.0	851.0
Wyoming	86.1	73.1	25.4	128.3	81.7	75.9	84.3	99.5	128.9	280.6	1010.9
Pacific	53.7	42.9	16.5	58.6	48.3	45.7	56.3	63.5	89.7	198.6	603.1
Alaska	106.5	96.5	62.9	99.0	109.2	123.0	168.8	116.6	160.2*	369.3*	580.7*
California	51.9	40.7	15.1	57.0	46.2	42.8	54.0	61.8	91.0	200.1	600.3
Hawaii	37.1	30.5	12.7	45.2	28.5	31.2	44.2	69.7	89.9	168.0	421.9
Oregon	64.2	57.5	23.2	75.2	60.7	60.9	66.7	71.1	83.8	175.4	549.9
Washington	56.5	43.9	17.4	57.2	52.3	50.0	57.6	64.6	85.9	206.7	668.2

Table 4   Death rates for all accidents, by age, white male:
United States, each geographic division and state, 1959-61
(E800-E962)

Geographic area	All ages	Under 5	5-14	15-24	25-34	35-44	45-54	55-64	65-74	75-84	85 & over
United States	69.7	42.2	24.6	92.4	67.4	60.3	71.4	83.8	116.1	238.1	612.8
New England	56.0	35.6	19.6	68.9	41.7	38.9	49.4	66.8	112.5	247.9	638.1
Connecticut	47.1	23.4	14.3	64.6	37.6	35.1	43.3	57.5	99.0	229.6	519.0
Maine	74.3	50.7	29.2	104.4	73.6	61.3	86.0	76.9	100.8	215.4	372.9
Massachusetts	56.6	32.4	18.6	60.0	35.9	36.8	47.3	74.5	128.1	278.3	787.6
New Hampshire	61.2	54.8	23.7	113.1	62.5	40.7	39.6	46.6	93.3	179.4	415.7
Rhode Island	42.8	53.0	19.7	41.4	28.0	30.5	33.4	37.3	75.7	214.3	570.9
Vermont	78.4	47.3	33.3	103.0	65.2	59.7	80.8	94.1	128.0	237.3	742.1
Middle Atlantic	54.2	30.9	19.4	67.5	42.6	38.2	50.7	68.8	108.4	233.3	581.2
New Jersey	47.8	33.7	18.6	62.0	35.8	29.4	45.2	65.2	92.1	215.3	614.8
New York	53.2	28.3	18.5	63.7	42.5	37.2	48.4	66.9	108.0	232.6	587.1
Pennsylvania	59.1	33.1	21.0	75.7	46.5	44.6	57.2	74.0	117.3	242.4	559.1
East North Central	64.9	36.7	23.6	89.7	58.9	51.5	62.1	81.4	118.5	246.1	599.6
Illinois	59.8	32.7	21.4	78.9	55.0	50.2	58.4	79.3	104.4	204.4	442.7
Indiana	74.8	43.6	27.1	100.6	71.6	61.9	73.0	85.3	122.7	284.5	728.5
Michigan	64.9	41.4	24.5	89.9	59.5	53.0	61.1	81.5	127.2	251.2	661.3
Ohio	62.8	32.1	23.0	82.9	56.2	45.7	61.5	82.9	122.3	266.4	626.8
Wisconsin	70.4	39.3	24.3	116.6	58.8	54.6	62.4	79.5	124.3	244.1	627.6
West North Central	77.6	44.1	27.0	104.6	72.2	64.9	77.9	88.8	122.0	240.8	688.9
Iowa	76.3	46.3	27.8	103.0	67.2	63.1	77.0	80.2	121.1	232.1	680.7
Kansas	79.1	45.7	27.8	109.8	77.3	63.8	77.1	90.1	119.3	228.9	751.4
Minnesota	72.2	39.4	26.2	100.0	61.2	63.9	72.6	85.2	124.5	241.8	687.7
Missouri	78.6	45.1	24.4	99.9	73.7	62.9	81.5	88.3	116.1	252.8	702.6
Nebraska	79.7	41.9	24.2	105.8	74.0	65.5	74.7	99.4	134.0	258.4	650.8
North Dakota	83.8	47.6	35.5	108.9	89.4	81.5	87.5	93.9	141.8	219.1	581.9
South Dakota	89.8	50.8	36.4	137.0	102.5	75.6	87.2	114.9	113.4	217.6	599.9
South Atlantic	73.6	46.1	28.1	96.9	78.2	73.2	80.4	87.7	102.7	214.4	551.4
Delaware	58.2	29.7	18.3	93.9	64.5	42.7	58.5	71.3	119.7	166.4*	643.7*
District of Columbia	74.0	52.7*	14.5*	57.2	40.3	68.9	90.3	76.4	149.8	236.2	512.2*
Florida	74.4	62.3	32.1	101.2	77.2	68.8	79.5	73.5	80.5	171.0	523.2
Georgia	78.6	45.0	30.0	103.3	86.9	83.5	90.8	92.3	115.1	238.8	551.8
Maryland	55.6	31.3	22.3	71.3	54.9	43.5	54.2	81.3	110.7	260.3	574.1
North Carolina	77.0	44.9	28.3	111.1	87.3	79.9	80.7	92.8	102.3	199.8	528.2
South Carolina	83.8	52.2	31.0	95.5	101.7	96.7	93.3	111.4	127.2	260.2	695.7
Virginia	68.4	40.6	25.0	84.0	69.8	67.3	76.3	88.5	113.4	245.0	584.1
West Virginia	87.4	45.8	31.1	118.0	89.8	101.5	103.8	105.8	111.7	225.8	514.2
East South Central	83.4	46.2	27.4	111.5	93.6	86.0	99.8	96.6	113.4	223.6	604.7
Alabama	86.1	45.1	27.6	113.3	108.6	92.0	102.3	104.9	117.7	211.2	583.4
Kentucky	85.9	47.2	26.0	115.2	90.0	80.9	109.1	98.7	125.2	239.4	715.0
Mississippi	93.7	51.9	30.1	121.8	104.4	108.5	116.6	99.1	124.6	249.7	416.8
Tennessee	74.6	43.5	27.5	101.8	80.4	76.8	82.1	87.3	92.8	203.6	578.3
West South Central	82.2	50.9	30.9	107.2	88.1	79.9	91.5	99.1	122.4	241.3	645.1
Arkansas	90.7	52.9	35.4	119.4	105.0	87.7	96.6	88.3	123.9	221.3	575.6
Louisiana	82.6	45.2	29.9	117.4	95.2	75.1	94.7	106.2	126.3	275.9	626.2
Oklahoma	90.4	58.3	32.2	105.8	85.4	78.9	112.7	105.0	133.0	229.8	662.3
Texas	78.7	50.6	30.2	103.1	84.5	80.2	84.1	97.7	117.5	242.7	660.1
Mountain	96.3	66.7	31.5	132.2	108.0	96.3	107.7	118.3	143.3	277.7	709.7
Arizona	90.6	71.4	28.7	126.9	104.4	92.5	110.8	102.5	123.7	219.1	612.0
Colorado	84.7	58.3	29.2	102.2	87.8	75.7	92.4	106.9	138.4	286.9	672.4
Idaho	104.3	80.9	39.1	141.3	100.8	96.2	117.0	124.2	164.3	260.1	846.5
Montana	113.7	63.4	35.9	185.1	131.0	117.4	111.1	132.4	148.3	265.0	670.7
Nevada	118.1	63.1	29.1	142.0	125.8	114.8	143.4	165.5	204.1	432.5	653.6*
New Mexico	107.2	70.1	35.1	149.2	150.5	124.1	105.2	136.2	147.3	305.9	717.2
Utah	77.9	58.2	25.2	103.0	78.0	80.5	104.6	98.3	125.9	276.5	733.4
Wyoming	125.8	88.3	38.7	218.0	135.0	122.2	124.0	147.8	159.6	319.0	933.6*
Pacific	74.6	48.8	22.3	93.6	76.9	69.1	82.6	91.5	125.0	238.1	589.7
Alaska	123.5	52.8	53.6	117.5	118.3	167.2	229.7	165.6	212.1*	535.0*	246.9*
California	71.2	46.9	20.4	91.3	73.1	63.1	77.8	88.0	125.8	239.8	564.3
Hawaii	57.9	30.6*	14.1*	76.7	47.2	60.1	63.5*	119.8*	124.8*	343.2*	508.9*
Oregon	93.1	64.1	29.8	124.9	99.0	99.3	103.2	106.2	121.2	212.8	692.6
Washington	78.7	51.1	25.3	87.7	84.7	77.1	86.1	95.4	122.1	240.3	637.3

Table 5   Death rates for all accidents, by age, white female:
United States, each geographic division and state, 1959-61
(E800-E962)

Geographic area	All ages	Under 5	5-14	15-24	25-34	35-44	45-54	55-64	65-74	75-84	85 & over
United States	31.1	31.2	10.0	19.3	14.0	15.5	21.5	29.2	58.6	195.2	674.5
New England	32.3	26.8	8.1	12.5	8.1	10.5	17.0	26.0	63.0	233.4	745.1
Connecticut	24.5	23.7	5.7	10.9	9.2	8.1	14.8	25.3	47.7	192.9	553.4
Maine	30.7	46.4	16.3	10.8	11.5	11.1	21.8	21.3	45.4	158.3	481.1
Massachusetts	37.2	22.7	7.3	12.4	6.6	10.9	17.1	27.6	78.9	279.2	914.1
New Hampshire	30.6	32.1	11.7	23.3	12.8*	15.0*	18.7	16.6*	38.7	173.1	538.9
Rhode Island	26.9	24.4	4.5*	8.9*	7.1*	8.2*	14.6	27.7	49.0	198.2	710.3
Vermont	35.4	44.0	12.1*	18.4*	9.0*	19.4*	23.1*	31.1*	38.6*	188.8	629.8
Middle Atlantic	26.8	23.6	7.2	12.8	8.6	10.3	15.3	24.8	58.6	205.1	603.9
New Jersey	24.8	25.1	6.1	11.4	8.0	10.0	14.4	19.8	56.0	204.2	618.4
New York	26.6	21.9	7.3	12.6	8.4	10.0	15.6	25.0	57.9	593.2	593.2
Pennsylvania	28.2	25.2	7.7	13.9	9.3	10.8	15.4	27.1	60.9	213.4	612.3
East North Central	30.3	26.0	9.8	18.3	13.6	14.6	20.3	29.9	59.9	195.3	698.1
Illinois	25.0	21.2	9.2	17.4	12.5	12.9	19.0	25.2	49.8	144.9	391.6
Indiana	35.7	31.5	12.5	20.1	14.7	16.4	24.2	33.5	66.1	217.3	845.0
Michigan	30.5	30.5	10.2	19.9	13.3	14.3	21.5	30.5	63.2	213.1	849.2
Ohio	32.4	22.5	9.1	15.5	14.9	15.7	19.0	33.6	67.0	228.8	813.6
Wisconsin	31.2	29.5	8.9	21.6	12.2	14.4	20.3	29.2	56.9	184.4	743.6
West North Central	34.3	30.3	11.0	21.5	14.8	15.0	21.7	29.2	56.1	183.7	741.4
Iowa	36.2	30.3	11.5	23.9	15.3	17.2	23.0	31.0	45.0	180.6	767.8
Kansas	36.3	33.8	12.3	21.5	16.4	13.6	21.4	30.7	64.3	170.4	822.0
Minnesota	30.9	28.0	10.7	19.6	11.9	14.5	21.9	31.7	54.1	170.9	732.9
Missouri	36.8	30.6	10.2	20.1	15.5	16.0	21.6	28.0	62.9	201.9	744.9
Nebraska	32.0	32.6	9.1	23.7	15.4	12.0	20.3	21.9	46.0	176.6	654.5
North Dakota	31.4	30.8	14.2	17.5	14.2*	20.0	21.6	31.3	67.6	209.0	572.7
South Dakota	30.7	25.9	10.8	30.1	17.8	9.6*	20.6	25.6	56.7	173.9	619.6
South Atlantic	29.5	35.4	10.8	19.6	14.8	17.2	23.4	28.4	54.5	183.2	601.2
Delaware	22.8	17.7*	9.1*	9.4*	3.7*	10.6*	19.0*	23.5*	58.1	174.6	601.9
District of Columbia	43.1	53.3*	6.2*	9.7*	8.2*	22.2*	24.2	36.0	73.3	238.7	552.1
Florida	31.2	41.7	8.8	22.2	15.4	18.8	27.9	28.4	44.2	157.9	547.9
Georgia	31.7	37.1	13.6	25.6	19.8	16.6	25.4	29.8	54.7	183.7	658.0
Maryland	25.6	23.8	9.7	12.7	8.5	14.4	20.5	26.7	63.8	200.6	508.9
North Carolina	27.5	37.1	10.8	22.3	13.4	17.5	21.0	30.7	53.3	164.7	517.2
South Carolina	32.8	44.2	15.4	20.2	21.2	24.3	24.8	32.1	59.5	204.0	666.3
Virginia	27.6	29.9	8.9	16.2	13.5	13.1	19.8	23.0	59.4	213.5	717.2
West Virginia	31.4	38.4	11.8	17.7	17.8	20.1	23.6	29.0	59.0	176.0	693.3
East South Central	33.4	41.4	12.7	22.6	17.2	17.2	23.0	29.8	57.5	197.7	742.4
Alabama	32.9	45.7	14.6	22.5	16.9	18.7	26.0	31.6	55.6	195.7	663.7
Kentucky	35.6	37.8	11.7	22.0	16.0	17.5	19.0	29.7	63.9	230.0	902.7
Mississippi	37.3	47.5	15.8	24.4	25.5	20.6	25.6	33.3	65.7	193.9	638.2
Tennessee	30.0	39.3	11.0	22.4	15.2	14.6	23.2	27.0	49.1	167.9	669.9
West South Central	33.6	38.7	12.1	24.4	16.8	20.8	25.4	31.8	57.2	200.8	695.5
Arkansas	36.5	49.4	13.1	30.9	11.1	21.6	22.5	31.1	53.9	191.5	708.3
Louisiana	31.5	34.0	11.1	24.5	17.1	15.7	20.0	34.2	60.6	215.9	808.8
Oklahoma	41.3	36.9	14.2	31.9	16.6	24.9	28.1	37.5	64.1	204.8	810.5
Texas	31.7	38.9	11.8	21.4	17.6	21.0	26.6	29.5	54.7	197.7	621.7
Mountain	37.5	47.3	14.1	30.9	21.8	21.7	34.0	37.9	70.2	193.4	790.8
Arizona	32.0	57.1	10.5	25.6	16.6	24.8	29.6	39.6	61.9	138.5	468.8
Colorado	38.0	34.8	15.7	26.8	20.9	20.8	33.9	39.8	58.5	195.9	777.4
Idaho	42.2	54.9	19.0	33.0	26.2	25.7	39.8	37.8	74.2	187.9	734.3
Montana	40.1	41.3	17.2	35.3	26.8	13.8*	41.0	26.0*	75.0	184.5	953.5
Nevada	51.9	80.3	20.6*	47.9	36.6	29.6*	46.4	57.3*	136.9	207.4*	1039.0*
New Mexico	34.1	53.4	10.6	35.5	19.7	18.6	32.7	31.7	70.2	213.5	840.3
Utah	35.6	39.1	12.4	30.1	20.1	19.5	27.1	36.4	82.2	233.0	917.6
Wyoming	42.1	53.4	12.9*	35.3	25.4*	27.1*	33.4*	48.2*	81.8	230.8	1011.6
Pacific	32.9	34.0	9.3	22.5	18.7	21.0	27.9	35.2	58.5	171.3	622.4
Alaska	30.9	44.6*	18.7*	27.1*	19.9*	28.5*	46.9*	24.7*	102.0*	217.9*	653.6*
California	33.3	32.9	8.8	22.2	19.5	21.1	28.4	35.9	61.2	174.8	631.8
Hawaii	20.2	23.6*	9.2*	12.2*	4.4*	17.5*	30.0*	58.0*	61.9*	121.2*	308.6*
Oregon	33.8	47.5	14.5	25.7	22.0	22.4	26.4	34.3	45.9	143.6	460.5
Washington	31.2	31.8	7.6	22.6	13.4	19.1	24.9	31.0	52.3	173.7	685.9

Table 6

Death rates for all accidents, by age, nonwhite male:
United States, each geographic division and state, 1959-61
(E800-E962)

Geographic area	All ages	Under 5	5-14	15-24	25-34	35-44	45-54	55-64	65-74	75-84	85 & over
United States	92.5	86.8	37.3	95.8	103.8	110.3	122.7	130.8	138.7	191.7	335.9
New England	80.9	88.9	38.2	68.1	65.8	94.9	103.6	85.2	192.4	299.5*	334.2*
Connecticut	78.8	74.8	40.6*	100.1	85.3	117.8	91.9*	11.1*	113.0*	135.2*	-
Maine	187.8*	64.0*	63.6*	108.0*	92.7*	612.7*	632.9*	282.5*	716.8*	952.4*	-
Massachusetts	82.4	109.1	42.6*	41.0*	55.9*	58.2*	100.8*	132.5*	240.1*	345.3*	634.9*
New Hampshire	23.1*	-	-	-	-	243.3*	-	-	-	-	-
Rhode Island	56.7*	80.3*	-	69.2*	20.4*	81.0*	98.9*	115.3*	78.2*	192.7*	-
Vermont	79.0*	-	-	-	-	-	-	-	-	2777.8*	-
Middle Atlantic	78.7	78.7	33.3	63.7	77.7	94.2	111.4	108.9	127.5	160.9	263.7
New Jersey	90.1	120.5	36.0	79.9	77.6	91.8	128.3	130.2	163.2	114.5*	244.2*
New York	75.9	63.0	31.8	61.9	83.4	96.2	105.9	102.8	112.5	148.7	212.9*
Pennsylvania	76.5	77.6	33.9	56.1	66.2	92.1	111.3	107.3	129.3	199.2	329.1*
East North Central	67.3	58.9	29.7	60.2	67.7	79.2	92.3	101.6	119.5	179.9	344.5
Illinois	64.3	59.5	25.8	56.9	70.1	74.4	92.1	94.9	99.0	157.3	281.3*
Indiana	77.6	67.6	30.9	88.9	66.5	84.8	96.4	120.3	129.9	282.3*	360.4*
Michigan	59.1	51.2	25.4	51.1	53.7	72.1	88.3	95.8	112.2	156.8*	329.5*
Ohio	73.9	60.8	37.9	56.8	75.7	92.1	91.7	105.2	134.8	194.8	446.6*
Wisconsin	79.2	66.8*	35.5*	102.1*	80.3*	65.8*	132.2*	151.8*	268.3*	-	-
West North Central	109.0	96.5	35.5	112.3	112.1	127.7	132.5	167.3	174.9	244.2	562.9
Iowa	73.2	49.0*	31.7*	119.7*	71.2*	61.6*	160.0*	60.9*	87.6*	113.4*	-
Kansas	70.0	59.3*	23.0*	76.9*	59.2*	84.4*	53.0*	79.9*	140.4*	202.5*	751.9*
Minnesota	135.1	77.5*	40.3*	195.8*	106.8*	228.2*	123.3*	346.1*	114.3*	199.0*	1515.2*
Missouri	99.2	106.8	31.1	69.1	81.5	114.1	114.8	167.2	189.3	263.4	485.4*
Nebraska	110.4	66.5*	24.3*	155.9*	98.8*	99.0*	245.8*	203.3*	165.8*	109.6*	1169.6*
North Dakota	223.2	162.6*	128.6*	220.6*	263.5*	304.1*	299.0*	662.3*	192.7*	456.6*	-
South Dakota	325.2	157.0*	84.5*	426.2	797.2	393.1*	596.5*	207.0*	317.5*	480.8*	-
South Atlantic	104.7	100.1	41.4	111.1	126.1	132.5	143.0	157.3	145.9	182.5	240.1
Delaware	101.2	64.8*	29.9*	109.9*	142.0*	110.6*	142.9*	164.1*	148.0*	128.2*	326.8*
District of Columbia	76.5	86.5	29.0	66.8	51.0	78.6	126.3	126.4	134.1	199.3*	525.5*
Florida	117.8	104.4	56.0	121.6	121.3	144.1	169.1	190.4	135.3	218.1	139.0*
Georgia	99.2	106.8	39.5	104.9	132.7	123.0	133.7	137.1	123.0	148.4	214.7*
Maryland	96.6	105.1	37.4	78.4	92.2	107.9	132.5	154.8	192.4	292.0	316.5*
North Carolina	108.3	107.8	36.4	125.9	148.2	149.7	131.8	153.2	177.2	160.3	204.2*
South Carolina	117.3	106.9	51.2	122.3	199.2	173.0	177.3	152.7	107.4	167.0	125.5*
Virginia	99.8	78.5	34.0	112.9	109.8	130.7	127.0	159.4	156.9	185.9	372.6*
West Virginia	107.9	43.4*	43.1*	90.7*	145.6*	103.2*	165.9	222.9	156.2*	118.0*	152.9*
East South Central	99.2	98.2	42.1	98.9	125.7	131.1	128.5	133.3	126.8	188.5	347.8
Alabama	101.1	88.0	43.2	107.0	137.2	128.0	134.3	157.2	138.1	146.0	341.8*
Kentucky	107.6	129.5	28.1*	110.6	105.1	133.8	116.5	126.1	137.7	281.9	319.0*
Mississippi	102.9	109.6	45.4	102.6	150.6	145.9	126.7	120.6	110.8	223.7	435.2
Tennessee	87.0	85.2	38.8	72.9	86.8	117.2	126.6	119.6	129.7	149.3	221.4*
West South Central	97.8	93.0	37.9	108.9	120.2	116.7	120.8	132.2	139.4	193.6	311.2
Arkansas	112.8	104.4	48.2	133.3	135.1	130.5	164.1	130.2	146.7	205.9	317.2*
Louisiana	93.6	80.4	33.8	124.4	133.0	111.0	99.2	125.2	130.7	196.0	385.9
Oklahoma	120.0	93.3	35.2	128.4	148.8	137.5	159.8	216.6	178.2	214.7*	437.3*
Texas	92.5	100.7	38.6	83.5	103.8	114.3	117.8	121.8	134.9	179.7	208.0*
Mountain	186.7	133.8	42.1	215.5	266.6	236.4	321.6	296.3	267.3	345.5	746.7*
Arizona	194.4	159.2	28.8*	214.5	291.5	279.7	354.3	297.2	322.9	187.5*	839.3*
Colorado	104.1	65.3*	24.2*	106.4*	110.5*	121.9*	167.0*	166.1*	229.2*	306.5*	749.1*
Idaho	214.7	221.6*	84.6*	287.7*	352.5*	220.4*	162.6*	219.3*	142.5*	508.9*	-
Montana	231.8	135.4*	60.9*	311.7*	362.3*	288.9*	261.6*	565.0*	159.1*	817.0*	724.6*
Nevada	175.2	126.1*	57.6*	207.9*	134.9*	252.9*	372.6*	249.9*	214.4*	350.9*	-
New Mexico	216.5	142.4	55.6*	240.2	381.6	278.9	409.6	401.6	163.4*	236.4*	590.0*
Utah	194.8	23.9*	83.4*	304.9*	267.7*	174.8*	272.3*	146.2*	375.6*	744.9*	1234.6*
Wyoming	172.8*	163.9*	-	113.2*	221.2*	171.4*	477.9*	-	775.2*	595.2*	2564.1*
Pacific	76.4	60.2	30.4	83.5	84.4	81.1	97.7	103.4	137.5	204.2	548.9
Alaska	231.7	240.0	165.9	177.6	330.0	287.2	309.4*	220.3*	169.8*	297.6*	-
California	70.9	52.3	24.5	76.9	71.7	81.4	97.2	100.8	143.2	187.5	533.3
Hawaii	52.5	33.1	20.3	63.5	53.1	40.4	61.6	82.6	122.8	199.8	531.2*
Oregon	139.2	137.1*	56.6*	181.8*	159.7*	131.8*	192.5*	100.5*	225.5*	214.4*	-
Washington	140.7	111.7	52.9*	142.0	207.8	153.0	166.7	205.6	92.4*	342.9*	1199.0*

Table 7 — Death rates for all accidents, by age, nonwhite female:
United States, each geographic division and state, 1959-61
(E800-E962)

Geographic area	All ages	Under 5	5-14	15-24	25-34	35-44	45-54	55-64	65-74	75-84	85 & over
United States	37.4	74.7	18.9	19.9	24.3	29.1	32.9	45.8	71.9	138.4	310.4
New England	33.5	55.1	29.6	16.6*	26.8*	24.2*	28.7*	21.3*	73.4*	111.8*	281.9*
Connecticut	30.5	54.1*	32.2*	18.9*	17.5*	17.0*	45.3*	10.8*	79.7*	54.6*	-
Maine	25.6*	67.8*	-	-	62.0*	-	-	-	-	-	-
Massachusetts	35.4	56.3*	29.0*	11.0*	29.0*	27.5*	18.2*	33.7*	72.1*	137.2*	486.6*
New Hampshire	29.2*	-	-	-	125.3*	-	-	-	-	-	-
Rhode Island	42.5*	59.5*	30.9*	43.7*	41.6*	55.1*	-	-	84.2*	165.0*	-
Vermont	-	-	-	-	-	-	-	-	-	-	-
Middle Atlantic	29.4	57.6	15.3	11.9	19.3	27.6	27.1	44.7	56.8	112.2	228.5
New Jersey	34.3	86.5	16.1	10.1*	26.6	30.8	24.7	39.8	46.7*	138.9*	207.6*
New York	27.0	51.8	11.6	15.1	14.6	27.4	29.7	40.2	55.9	83.1	265.0*
Pennsylvania	30.7	48.5	20.4	7.0*	24.1	26.0	23.9	54.5	63.6	137.9	194.7*
East North Central	27.2	51.1	13.6	18.6	19.8	19.6	23.3	23.7	53.8	108.2	290.7
Illinois	25.2	58.6	15.6	16.2	15.7	17.4	16.9	23.6	44.3	69.3*	163.0*
Indiana	32.2	71.7	7.6*	12.5*	25.8*	14.6*	41.3*	42.2*	58.1*	143.1*	330.0*
Michigan	23.7	36.8	11.9	15.0	20.9	21.4	17.1*	40.6	61.6	98.9*	190.5*
Ohio	30.6	44.9	13.7	27.4	21.2	22.6	28.9	38.2	59.9	146.2	469.5*
Wisconsin	35.1	59.0*	23.5*	19.2*	29.4*	18.9*	51.8*	35.7*	32.6*	178.7*	1058.2*
West North Central	50.6	84.5	20.9	31.1	34.8	37.2	53.8	52.0	84.2	223.9	431.9
Iowa	56.6	128.3*	31.5*	30.7*	-	79.5*	74.2*	31.6*	89.0*	-	374.5*
Kansas	40.7	68.5*	9.9*	9.4*	29.1*	53.0*	72.8*	41.5*	58.9*	110.0*	222.2*
Minnesota	62.5	70.5*	6.7*	54.4*	64.8*	85.1*	61.6*	-	215.1*	484.5*	416.7*
Missouri	45.7	88.3	20.6	16.1*	26.5	24.5*	35.2	58.0	82.4	242.3	474.4*
Nebraska	53.3	68.1*	33.3*	54.3*	48.5*	15.7*	65.2*	28.5*	87.8*	101.3*	1052.6*
North Dakota	110.5	80.5*	73.9*	100.2*	130.0*	173.6*	245.7*	117.0*	205.8*	-	-
South Dakota	105.6	89.5*	26.7*	181.8*	115.3*	53.7*	253.3*	101.3*	-	732.6*	-
South Atlantic	40.4	85.1	21.5	18.5	27.3	32.3	36.0	53.2	77.1	125.3	259.3
Delaware	37.6	36.1*	29.5*	23.5*	23.4*	65.6*	31.7*	48.2*	-	141.5*	617.3*
District of Columbia	29.6	82.7	11.1*	6.6*	14.5*	22.0	23.2*	28.4*	82.2*	127.1*	325.0*
Florida	44.1	82.6	24.7	23.1	32.1	36.0	47.0	66.2	70.7	119.9	187.8*
Georgia	44.4	90.6	22.7	16.4	30.0	40.9	38.0	78.2	68.1	124.6	224.6*
Maryland	36.5	68.3	17.2	20.8	26.3	37.4	32.5	31.6*	51.4*	220.0	357.6*
North Carolina	38.9	93.7	21.8	16.1	28.8	27.8	27.4	43.6	80.5	93.0	346.6
South Carolina	47.9	103.4	31.4	27.5	31.5	30.0	44.4	62.3	98.6	67.3*	111.0*
Virginia	32.9	61.3	11.1	13.6	22.1	26.8	37.4	35.0	83.0	161.0	290.2*
West Virginia	44.5	107.1*	12.6*	27.4*	28.1*	24.7*	18.3*	55.8*	105.6*	195.9*	330.0*
East South Central	43.9	90.9	21.7	21.3	27.0	30.2	34.2	41.1	73.9	167.2	416.3
Alabama	43.0	90.7	21.9	21.0	22.5	30.8	30.1	47.0	76.1	163.6	419.1
Kentucky	46.9	84.3	13.4*	21.1*	25.1*	29.8*	30.0*	58.8*	65.3*	201.5*	801.1*
Mississippi	47.7	107.6	27.1	24.9	24.8	29.9	30.1	39.5	67.6	170.0	426.9
Tennessee	38.2	64.6	14.1	15.5	37.5	30.0	47.3	27.2	83.8	151.8	221.0*
West South Central	43.4	88.3	20.2	23.7	25.3	30.4	36.1	52.0	84.6	147.3	274.0
Arkansas	49.4	109.2	29.5	19.2*	23.2*	21.9*	30.9*	46.9	91.1	191.6	260.6*
Louisiana	40.3	77.6	17.1	19.9	22.5	26.5	38.6	52.6	88.4	121.5	439.2
Oklahoma	57.2	108.5	22.8*	31.9*	59.6	40.8*	46.2*	54.0*	102.2	170.1*	289.4*
Texas	41.7	87.2	19.3	27.2	22.6	34.1	33.9	53.1	74.8	146.7	127.8*
Mountain	72.1	122.8	18.5	63.9	61.4	87.1	78.9	75.7*	92.0*	289.1*	730.7*
Arizona	75.7	118.0	17.4*	62.2	81.1	82.9*	83.7*	99.3*	95.3*	463.0*	734.2*
Colorado	34.1	76.2*	6.1*	36.3*	36.8*	28.3*	32.8*	21.4*	32.6	-	311.5*
Idaho	71.1*	86.9*	53.2*	102.9*	52.3*	63.7*	-	-	-	456.6*	1449.3*
Montana	142.9	244.6*	41.5*	106.0*	114.9*	303.9*	177.1*	189.0*	99.5*	198.4*	-
Nevada	100.5	176.3*	28.5*	109.6*	77.3*	143.4*	80.4*	-	121.2*	438.6*	1010.1*
New Mexico	57.3	99.0	15.7*	40.4*	38.1*	95.3*	68.6*	87.6*	42.4*	224.5*	775.2*
Utah	82.6	178.1*	16.0*	25.7*	55.7*	34.3*	137.2*	84.0*	429.2*	432.9*	1960.8*
Wyoming	105.4*	105.2*	-	340.1*	-	-	149.5*	-	300.3*	854.7*	4761.9*
Pacific	27.7	47.4	14.7	19.2	18.1	25.2	28.7	35.7	60.5	114.6	323.3
Alaska	123.6	197.3	87.6*	74.2*	141.5*	116.9*	134.5*	-	74.6*	165.8*	1785.7*
California	25.5	41.9	12.4	16.1	15.5	24.1	29.2	36.3	62.4	113.4	274.0*
Hawaii	16.1	30.9*	5.5*	10.8*	7.4*	12.3*	12.2*	34.8*	46.8	91.3*	277.8*
Oregon	73.3	84.8*	65.4*	79.7*	51.0*	54.6*	85.2*	137.0*	117.4*	-	-
Washington	41.9	63.9*	20.9*	41.5*	29.7*	55.0*	28.6*	-	70.7*	276.6*	476.2*

Table 8   Age-adjusted death rates for all accidents, by color and sex:
United States, each geographic division and state, 1959-61
(E800-E962)

Geographic area	Total			White			Nonwhite		
	Total	Male	Female	Total	Male	Female	Total	Male	Female
United States	49.4	73.3	26.4	47.3	70.2	25.1	65.5	98.6	34.9
New England	37.8	54.3	22.1	37.3	53.5	21.8	57.4	84.1	31.5
Connecticut	33.4	48.7	19.0	32.3	46.9	18.4	54.0	80.7	29.4
Maine	48.6	75.2	22.3	48.2	74.4	22.3	160.3	283.4*	14.4*
Massachusetts	37.8	53.0	23.6	37.3	52.3	23.3	56.7	82.1	32.0
New Hampshire	42.2	61.6	22.9	42.2	61.9	22.8	28.1*	33.9*	20.3*
Rhode Island	29.6	40.1	18.9	29.0	39.7	18.3	50.1	61.6*	39.3*
Vermont	50.1	76.4	25.1	50.2	76.4	25.1	23.1*	48.1*	-
Middle Atlantic	37.4	55.1	21.0	35.8	52.6	20.1	52.8	80.7	28.3
New Jersey	35.5	51.2	20.4	33.0	47.4	19.0	60.0	91.4	31.2
New York	36.4	53.5	20.6	34.8	51.0	19.8	50.2	77.9	26.6
Pennsylvania	40.0	59.4	22.0	38.9	57.8	21.2	52.4	78.1	29.3
East North Central	44.9	66.1	24.6	44.4	65.5	24.3	48.2	71.5	26.4
Illinois	40.3	60.5	21.0	39.6	59.5	20.5	44.4	68.0	22.9
Indiana	51.2	75.4	28.0	50.9	74.9	27.8	55.2	82.4	29.9
Michigan	46.1	66.8	26.1	46.1	66.9	26.0	43.7	63.6	24.6
Ohio	44.5	64.4	25.8	43.7	63.2	25.1	53.2	77.1	30.6
Wisconsin	47.9	71.7	24.8	47.5	71.3	24.5	64.6	92.8	36.1
West North Central	51.6	77.6	26.4	50.4	76.1	25.5	78.5	113.2	46.2
Iowa	49.8	74.1	26.4	49.6	74.0	26.2	64.1	81.2	48.5
Kansas	52.1	77.4	27.1	52.0	77.9	26.5	53.5	68.8	37.8
Minnesota	48.4	73.0	24.8	47.7	72.1	24.3	110.4	153.1	65.8
Missouri	51.5	77.1	27.3	50.0	75.2	25.9	66.5	97.2	39.4
Nebraska	51.2	78.5	24.5	50.2	77.3	23.8	88.0	126.0	49.6
North Dakota	59.3	88.7	28.5	56.7	85.6	26.6	199.5	264.9	130.7
South Dakota	67.1	104.3	29.2	59.4	92.7	25.5	259.6	399.1	121.4
South Atlantic	55.7	83.8	28.5	50.3	75.6	25.5	74.3	114.3	37.7
Delaware	44.3	68.3	21.0	39.7	62.0	18.3	72.9	108.9	36.8
District of Columbia	48.2	72.0	27.8	42.7	62.4	25.9	51.6	79.3	27.0
Florida	55.5	83.1	28.9	49.8	74.5	25.9	82.8	125.4	41.9
Georgia	59.9	89.2	32.2	55.1	82.5	28.4	72.4	108.5	41.2
Maryland	44.5	65.6	24.2	39.8	58.6	21.7	68.3	102.1	35.3
North Carolina	58.5	90.0	28.2	52.7	80.6	25.2	76.9	122.1	35.7
South Carolina	68.8	103.5	35.7	59.7	89.2	30.4	87.4	137.3	44.2
Virginia	51.7	78.2	25.3	47.3	70.8	23.6	69.1	108.1	31.3
West Virginia	58.6	91.7	27.5	57.8	90.5	26.9	73.0	112.7	39.6
East South Central	59.8	90.6	30.6	56.7	86.3	28.1	70.3	107.6	38.2
Alabama	63.0	96.5	31.8	59.2	90.7	29.0	71.8	112.3	37.5
Kentucky	58.9	89.3	28.9	57.9	87.9	28.2	71.3	106.9	37.9
Mississippi	68.4	103.3	35.8	64.0	96.6	31.9	74.0	114.7	39.8
Tennessee	52.3	79.0	27.3	50.5	76.6	25.6	61.4	90.8	35.5
West South Central	58.8	87.9	30.7	56.5	84.8	28.9	70.0	105.0	38.8
Arkansas	63.7	97.0	32.2	59.8	91.0	29.6	77.6	121.9	39.6
Louisiana	60.6	92.6	30.7	57.4	88.2	28.0	68.0	104.2	36.3
Oklahoma	62.5	91.5	34.5	60.0	88.1	32.5	88.5	129.5	51.9
Texas	56.2	83.9	29.4	54.8	82.2	28.0	65.9	96.2	38.2
Mountain	71.5	106.6	36.1	68.0	101.5	34.3	146.3	215.5	73.1
Arizona	71.6	108.0	35.0	63.4	96.2	30.5	156.3	229.0	80.4
Colorado	59.1	86.7	32.2	58.7	85.9	32.1	73.5	115.0	31.7
Idaho	74.1	109.0	38.5	72.9	107.1	38.0	149.2	224.3	63.7*
Montana	82.5	124.6	39.0	78.1	119.7	35.3	216.8	276.6	150.4
Nevada	92.5	126.4	55.2	88.1	121.4	51.7	149.8	194.6	96.4
New Mexico	82.1	127.6	35.9	76.4	118.0	34.1	160.3	259.1	60.4
Utah	60.4	87.2	34.1	58.7	84.6	33.3	157.2	217.6	92.0
Wyoming	89.0	135.3	40.8	87.7	134.4	39.2	165.8	204.0*	129.6*
Pacific	52.2	76.2	28.1	51.8	75.6	28.0	56.1	81.6	28.2
Alaska	116.0	158.8	54.5	97.8	137.6	36.8	182.1	240.2	109.9
California	50.5	72.8	28.2	50.3	72.4	28.2	52.1	76.4	26.3
Hawaii	41.0	59.2	18.9	46.6	65.2	23.0	38.3	56.6	17.1
Oregon	62.7	96.0	30.4	61.7	94.9	29.5	110.3	143.0	74.8
Washington	53.8	81.1	26.2	52.1	78.4	25.6	99.7	148.4	41.3

Table 9   Death rates for all accidents and specified types of accidents:
United States, each geographic division and state, 1959-61

Geographic area	All accidents (E800-E962)	Motor-vehicle (E810-E835)	Falls (E900-E904)	Machinery (E912)	Fire and explosion (E916)	Firearm (E919)	Inhalation and ingestion (E921,E922)	Drowning (E929)
United States	51.7	21.2	10.5	1.1	4.0	1.3	1.3	2.9
New England	44.2	13.0	15.6	0.5	3.5	0.6	1.3	2.5
Connecticut	36.4	11.7	11.3	0.4	2.9	0.4	1.2	2.2
Maine	52.6	17.5	10.1	1.0	6.2	1.9	1.6	3.5
Massachusetts	46.8	12.2	19.9	0.4	3.3	0.4	1.2	2.4
New Hampshire	45.5	17.1	9.8	0.8*	4.1	0.9*	0.9*	3.1
Rhode Island	35.1	8.9	13.1	0.2*	3.2	0.2*	2.1	1.7
Vermont	56.5	22.6	13.9	2.1	4.1	1.6*	1.4*	3.0
Middle Atlantic	41.2	14.0	12.6	0.6	3.1	0.5	1.0	2.2
New Jersey	38.3	12.8	11.4	0.5	3.1	0.4	1.2	2.4
New York	40.4	13.5	13.1	0.5	3.1	0.5	0.9	2.4
Pennsylvania	44.0	15.3	12.4	0.8	3.1	0.7	1.0	1.9
East North Central	47.3	20.2	10.9	1.1	3.2	0.8	1.0	2.3
Illinois	42.3	17.3	8.6	1.0	3.3	0.9	0.7	2.3
Indiana	55.0	24.4	12.8	1.3	3.6	0.9	1.0	2.3
Michigan	47.0	21.2	10.3	0.9	3.1	0.6	1.4	2.5
Ohio	47.7	19.4	12.6	1.0	3.1	0.7	0.9	2.2
Wisconsin	50.8	22.5	11.5	1.6	2.7	1.0	1.1	2.3
West North Central	56.7	24.1	12.7	2.3	3.5	1.3	1.2	2.4
Iowa	56.0	24.6	13.2	2.4	2.6	0.7	1.0	2.2
Kansas	57.5	25.1	11.9	2.6	3.6	1.6	1.3	2.4
Minnesota	52.0	22.1	11.4	1.8	2.7	1.2	1.3	2.5
Missouri	58.5	23.3	14.4	1.9	4.6	1.4	1.2	2.3
Nebraska	56.4	23.3	13.3	2.8	3.0	1.3	1.0	2.3
North Dakota	60.4	26.2	10.3	3.6	4.2	2.2	1.2	3.4
South Dakota	66.9	33.5	9.4	3.2	3.3	2.1	1.4	3.0
South Atlantic	56.0	23.1	7.9	1.0	5.3	1.9	1.6	3.9
Delaware	44.4	17.0	7.9	0.6*	4.9	1.0*	1.4*	3.6
District of Columbia	54.4	12.3	17.2	0.2*	5.6	0.8*	3.8	2.8
Florida	57.4	24.2	7.5	0.9	4.1	1.6	1.5	5.7
Georgia	59.3	25.5	6.9	1.1	6.2	2.7	1.7	3.6
Maryland	44.8	16.3	9.5	0.8	4.4	0.8	1.5	2.6
North Carolina	57.2	27.9	5.7	1.0	5.2	1.8	1.8	3.4
South Carolina	66.3	28.1	6.1	1.1	7.7	3.5	1.9	4.9
Virginia	51.7	19.8	8.9	1.2	4.9	1.5	1.4	3.2
West Virginia	59.8	20.3	10.2	1.3	5.8	2.2	1.0	3.5
East South Central	60.8	25.8	8.3	1.3	6.8	2.4	1.4	3.2
Alabama	62.6	28.5	6.5	1.3	7.2	2.3	1.4	3.2
Kentucky	61.8	24.5	12.6	1.3	5.4	2.0	1.4	3.0
Mississippi	69.1	27.3	6.1	1.6	10.2	4.1	1.6	5.1
Tennessee	53.4	23.3	7.8	1.3	5.6	1.7	1.4	2.4
West South Central	59.7	25.9	7.8	1.3	5.9	2.2	1.5	3.6
Arkansas	67.0	27.0	7.9	2.0	8.3	3.1	1.5	3.7
Louisiana	59.7	24.1	8.1	1.1	6.5	2.2	1.3	4.1
Oklahoma	67.6	29.5	11.7	1.5	6.0	2.1	1.3	2.9
Texas	56.5	25.5	6.7	1.1	5.3	2.0	1.6	3.5
Mountain	70.2	32.4	9.5	1.8	3.3	2.7	2.2	3.9
Arizona	69.0	33.2	6.0	1.0	4.2	2.4	2.3	4.9
Colorado	61.4	25.5	12.5	1.5	2.3	2.0	2.3	2.6
Idaho	74.7	33.7	10.5	2.9	2.7	3.3	1.3	6.1
Montana	81.5	36.4	10.9	3.0	3.4	4.0	1.6	5.8
Nevada	90.2	46.9	9.1	0.8*	4.4	3.0	2.3	3.9
New Mexico	76.9	38.5	6.9	1.8	4.3	2.9	2.5	3.6
Utah	58.3	27.1	9.1	1.5	2.2	2.7	2.0	3.0
Wyoming	86.1	40.1	11.5	4.0	4.3	3.6	3.3	3.0
Pacific	53.7	24.5	9.2	0.9	3.2	1.0	1.6	3.1
Alaska	106.7	15.8	4.4	2.1*	13.0	6.5	4.0	11.9
California	51.9	25.1	9.3	0.7	3.0	0.8	1.5	2.6
Hawaii	37.1	15.2	3.5	1.2	1.8	0.5*	1.4	5.0
Oregon	64.2	28.0	8.5	2.0	3.9	1.9	2.5	4.6
Washington	56.5	22.1	10.9	1.3	3.3	1.1	1.7	3.9

Table 10   Death rates for all accidents and specified types of accidents,
                by color and sex: United States, 1959-61

Type of accident	Total			White			Nonwhite		
	Total	Male	Female	Total	Male	Female	Total	Male	Female
All accidents (E800-E962)	51.7	72.3	31.8	50.1	69.7	31.1	64.2	92.6	37.4
Railway (E800-E802)	0.6	1.0	0.1	0.5	0.9	0.1	1.1	2.0	0.2
Motor-vehicle (E810-E835)	21.2	31.8	11.0	21.1	31.5	11.1	21.9	34.2	10.2
Traffic (E810-E825)	20.7	30.9	10.7	20.6	30.6	10.8	21.4	33.4	10.0
Involving collision with train (E810)	0.7	1.1	0.4	0.7	1.1	·0.4	0.5	0.8	0.3
To pedestrian (E812)	4.0	5.9	2.2	3.7	5.4	2.1	6.4	9.6	3.4
Nontraffic (E830-E835)	0.6	0.8	0.3	0.6	0.9	0.3	0.5	0.8	0.2
Water-transport (E850-E858)	0.8	1.6	0.1	0.8	1.5	0.1	1.0	2.0	0.1
Aircraft (E860-E866)	0.8	1.4	0.2	0.9	1.6	0.2	0.1	0.2	0.0*
Poisoning by solid and liquid substances (E870-E888)	1.0	1.2	0.7	0.8	1.0	0.6	2.1	2.8	1.5
Poisoning by gases and vapors (E890-E895)	0.7	1.0	0.4	0.6	1.0	0.3	0.8	1.1	0.6
Falls (E900-E904)	10.5	10.5	10.5	11.0	10.8	11.2	6.7	8.8	4.7
One level to another (E900-E902)	3.3	4.4	2.3	3.3	4.4	2.3	3.2	4.7	1.7
On same level (E903)	2.1	1.8	2.3	2.2	1.9	2.5	0.9	1.0	0.7
Unspecified falls (E904)	5.1	4.4	5.9	5.4	4.5	6.3	2.6	3.1	2.2
Blow from falling or projected object (E910)	0.8	1.5	0.1	0.8	1.5	0.1	0.9	1.8	0.1
Machinery (E912)	1.1	2.1	0.1	1.1	2.2	0.1	0.9	1.8	0.1
Electric current (E914)	0.6	1.0	0.1	0.6	1.1	0.1	0.4	0.8	0.1
Fire and explosion (E916)	4.0	4.6	3.4	3.2	3.8	2.5	10.7	11.0	10.4
Firearm (E919)	1.3	2.2	0.3	1.2	2.1	0.3	2.0	3.3	0.8
Inhalation and ingestion causing obstruction or suffocation (E921, E922)	1.3	1.6	1.0	1.2	1.5	0.9	2.3	2.7	1.9
Drowning (E929)	2.9	4.9	0.9	2.6	4.3	0.9	5.3	9.8	1.1

Table 11 Death rates for all accidents and specified types of accidents, by color and sex, for metropolitan and nonmetropolitan counties: United States, 1959-61

Type of accident	White					Nonwhite				
		Metropolitan counties			Non-metro-politan counties		Metropolitan counties			Non-metro-politan counties
	Total	Total	with central city	without central city		Total	Total	with central city	without central city	
Both sexes										
All accidents (E800-E962)	50.1	43.1	44.5	37.5	62.2	64.2	53.8	53.1	60.8	83.2
Motor-vehicle traffic to pedestrian (E812)	3.7	3.9	4.1	2.9	3.4	6.4	5.9	5.9	5.3	7.4
Motor-vehicle traffic excluding pedestrian (E810,E811,E813-E835)	17.4	13.2	13.3	12.9	24.8	15.5	11.6	11.1	18.1	22.4
Falls (E900-E904)	11.0	11.1	11.9	8.1	10.8	6.7	7.8	8.0	5.5	4.6
Fire and explosion (E916)	3.2	2.7	2.8	2.3	4.0	10.7	8.1	7.9	10.3	15.3
Drowning (E929)	2.6	2.3	2.3	2.0	3.1	5.3	4.3	4.3	4.4	7.1
Male										
All accidents	69.7	58.4	60.3	51.2	88.7	92.5	77.5	76.4	89.1	119.1
Motor-vehicle traffic to pedestrian	5.4	5.6	6.0	4.2	5.1	9.6	8.7	8.8	8.1	11.3
Motor-vehicle traffic excluding pedestrian	26.1	19.4	19.5	18.9	37.3	24.6	18.3	17.3	28.7	35.7
Falls	10.8	11.2	12.0	7.8	10.1	8.8	10.7	11.1	6.8	5.3
Fire and explosion	3.8	3.2	3.3	2.8	4.9	10.9	8.8	8.5	11.9	14.8
Drowning	4.3	3.8	4.0	3.3	5.1	9.8	8.0	8.0	8.2	12.9
Female										
All accidents	31.1	28.4	29.5	24.1	35.7	37.4	31.5	31.3	33.6	48.3
Motor-vehicle traffic to pedestrian	2.1	2.2	2.4	1.7	1.8	3.4	3.2	3.3	2.6	3.7
Motor-vehicle traffic excluding pedestrian	9.0	7.2	7.2	7.0	12.2	6.8	5.5	5.2	7.8	9.4
Falls	11.2	11.1	11.8	8.4	11.5	4.7	5.1	5.2	4.3	3.9
Fire and explosion	2.5	2.2	2.3	1.9	3.1	10.4	7.6	7.5	8.8	15.7
Drowning	0.9	0.8	0.8	0.7	1.0	1.1	0.9	0.9	0.8	1.4

Table 12   Death rates for all accidents and specified types of accidents,
white persons, by age and nativity: United States, 1959-61

Type of accident and nativity	All ages	Under 5	5-14	15-24	25-34	35-44	45-54	55-64	65-74	75-84	85 & over
All accidents (E800-E962)	50.1	36.8	17.4	55.5	40.3	37.5	45.8	55.2	86.6	220.7	700.3
Native	47.3	36.4	17.2	54.9	39.7	37.2	45.6	54.9	83.3	212.9	686.2
Foreign	83.3	69.0	20.0	55.2	38.2	30.9	37.0	49.9	92.5	236.4	715.7
Motor-vehicle traffic to pedestrian (E812)	3.7	3.3	3.3	1.6	1.2	1.7	2.8	5.4	10.6	19.8	21.2
Native	3.2	3.3	3.3	1.6	1.1	1.6	2.7	4.8	8.5	16.2	17.5
Foreign	10.8	11.3	4.8	2.5	2.3	2.4	3.9	7.9	17.7	31.0	34.2
Motor-vehicle traffic excluding pedestrian (E810, E811, E813-E835)	17.4	6.0	4.4	37.1	22.5	16.9	17.7	18.7	21.5	24.4	19.0
Native	17.4	5.8	4.3	36.9	22.3	16.9	17.9	19.5	23.0	25.9	20.3
Foreign	14.4	16.1	3.7	30.7	19.6	13.3	11.7	12.3	14.1	17.0	12.7
Falls (E900-E904)	11.0	2.0	0.6	1.1	1.4	2.6	5.4	10.6	30.6	135.2	582.5
Native	9.2	1.9	0.5	1.1	1.3	2.5	5.2	10.0	28.4	130.5	573.8
Foreign	36.8	6.9	1.0	1.4	1.5	2.7	6.2	12.7	36.9	145.9	585.2
Fire and explosion (E916)	3.2	3.9	1.5	1.1	1.9	2.4	3.6	3.9	6.6	15.0	27.9
Native	3.0	3.8	1.5	1.0	1.9	2.4	3.7	4.0	6.6	14.9	26.9
Foreign	4.6	6.6	1.1	1.4	1.4	1.3	2.6	2.9	5.8	14.2	28.4
Drowning (E929)	2.6	3.9	3.1	4.0	1.7	1.6	1.8	1.9	2.0	2.0	2.9
Native	2.5	3.8	3.0	3.8	1.7	1.5	1.6	1.7	1.6	1.4	1.9
Foreign	3.0	10.9	5.1	5.8	2.6	1.4	2.0	2.1	3.3	4.0	6.8

Table 13   Death rates for all accidents and specified types of accidents,
nonwhite persons, by race: United States, 1959-61

Type of accident	Total	Negro	Indian	Chinese	Japanese	Other
All accidents (E800-E962)	64.2	63.5	141.9	28.2	27.0	55.4
Motor-vehicle (E810-E835)	21.9	20.9	68.7	13.3	11.2	22.2
Traffic to pedestrian (E812)	6.4	6.2	17.6	4.2	3.1	5.2
Excluding pedestrian traffic						
(E810, E811, E813-E835)	15.5	14.7	51.1	9.1	8.1	17.0
Poisoning by solid and liquid sub-stances (E870-E888)	2.1	2.2	3.2	0.4*	0.3*	1.0*
Poisoning by gases and vapors (E890-E895)	0.8	0.9	1.3	0.4*	0.1*	0.2*
Falls (E900-E904)	6.7	6.8	8.5	4.7	3.5	4.7
Blow from falling or projected object (E910)	0.9	0.9	1.5	0.1*	0.1*	0.7*
Machinery (E912)	0.9	0.9	1.3	-	0.8*	1.3*
Electric current (E914)	0.4	0.5	0.4*	0.1*	0.2*	0.6*
Fire and explosion (E916)	10.7	11.1	12.6	1.1*	0.9*	4.2
Firearm (E919)	2.0	2.0	3.6	-	0.4*	0.8*
Inhalation and ingestion causing obstruction or suffocation(E921,E922)	2.3	2.3	3.9	1.0*	0.8*	2.0
Drowning (E929)	5.3	5.2	12.3	2.1*	3.7	5.8

Table 14

Age-adjusted death rates for all accidents
and specified types of accidents, persons age 15 and over,
by sex and marital status: United States, 1959-61

Marital status	All accidents (E800-E962)	Motor-vehicle traffic to pedestrian (E812)	Motor-vehicle excluding pedestrian traffic (E810, E811, E813-E835)	Falls (E900-E904)	Fire and explosion (E916)	Drowning (E929)
Both sexes, total	57.5	3.6	23.8	10.2	3.6	2.7
Single	86.5	7.7	29.3	17.0	6.1	5.2
Married	44.5	2.5	19.3	7.3	2.5	1.4
Widowed	102.4	4.8	52.0	12.2	9.8	4.3
Divorced	131.4	10.1	56.8	20.0	11.0	5.7
Males, total	87.5	5.7	37.3	11.8	4.6	4.9
Single	129.9	12.9	43.3	22.1	9.2	8.8
Married	71.2	3.8	32.2	8.7	3.1	3.0
Widowed	236.6	12.6	114.0	22.1	19.7	11.5
Divorced	240.0	18.1	103.9	32.5	18.6	11.7
Females, total	28.8	1.7	10.9	8.5	2.6	0.6
Single	33.9	2.5	9.5	11.3	3.1	0.8
Married	24.3	1.2	10.3	6.4	2.1	0.4
Widowed	69.3	3.0	36.3	10.0	7.3	2.6
Divorced	58.9	3.8	28.2	11.0	5.2	1.6

Table 15   Percent distribution of deaths from all accidents and specified types of accidents, by month of occurrence: United States 1959-61

Type of accident	Total	\multicolumn{13}{c}{Month of occurrence}
		Jan.	Feb.	Mar.	Apr.	May	June	July	Aug.	Sep.	Oct.	Nov.	Dec.
All accidents (E800-E962)	100.0	8.2	7.1	7.8	7.5	8.4	8.6	9.2	8.8	8.2	8.5	8.5	9.3
Railway (E800-E802)	100.0	6.4	5.8	8.1	7.3	8.9	10.1	10.6	9.7	9.3	9.3	7.5	6.9
Motor-vehicle (E810-E835)	100.0	7.3	6.2	7.0	7.5	8.3	8.4	8.9	9.2	8.9	9.5	9.2	9.6
Traffic (E810-E825)	100.0	7.3	6.3	7.0	7.4	8.3	8.3	8.8	9.1	8.8	9.5	9.3	9.7
Involving collision with train (E810)	100.0	12.9	8.5	9.0	6.7	6.1	7.8	5.6	5.7	5.9	8.0	10.8	12.9
To pedestrian (E812)	100.0	8.5	7.5	7.5	7.6	7.5	7.1	7.1	7.6	8.5	10.1	10.2	10.8
Involving two or more vehicles (E816)	100.0	7.0	6.3	7.3	7.2	8.2	8.1	9.0	9.6	8.7	9.3	9.2	9.9
Involving running off roadway (E823)	100.0	7.1	5.9	6.5	8.1	9.1	8.4	9.0	9.1	9.0	9.5	9.2	9.2
Nontraffic (E830-E835)	100.0	5.2	3.8	6.8	8.0	9.9	11.5	10.6	11.6	10.5	8.7	7.6	5.8
Water-transport (E850-E858)	100.0	3.2	3.8	5.6	8.6	14.2	13.1	16.0	13.0	7.3	6.2	5.5	3.5
Aircraft (E860-E866)	100.0	9.6	7.2	7.9	7.0	8.1	8.1	8.0	7.2	10.9	9.5	8.0	8.6
Poisoning by solid and liquid substances (E870-E888)	100.0	8.2	7.3	8.1	8.1	9.6	8.1	8.9	8.6	8.2	7.7	8.4	8.9
Poisoning by gases and vapors (E890-E895)	100.0	17.5	12.0	11.4	6.1	4.9	2.6	3.0	3.0	3.1	7.3	11.8	17.2
Falls (E900-E904)	100.0	9.1	8.2	8.5	7.6	8.2	8.2	8.2	8.1	8.0	8.4	8.3	9.2
One level to another (E900-E902)	100.0	7.9	7.1	7.3	7.5	8.6	8.8	9.2	9.0	8.8	8.8	8.5	8.5
On same level (E903)	100.0	10.5	9.4	9.6	7.5	8.2	7.5	7.2	7.4	7.5	7.7	7.9	9.7
Unspecified (E904)	100.0	9.3	8.4	8.7	7.8	7.9	8.2	7.9	7.8	7.7	8.4	8.3	9.5
Blow from falling or projected object (E910)	100.0	7.3	7.7	8.3	8.4	8.9	8.0	8.9	9.4	8.4	8.5	8.9	7.3
Machinery (E912)	100.0	4.6	5.5	6.6	8.9	10.6	10.1	10.0	10.6	10.0	9.5	7.7	6.0
Electric current (E914)	100.0	3.5	4.3	5.2	6.4	7.9	11.9	15.5	15.2	12.7	8.1	5.6	3.5
Fire and explosion (E916)	100.0	14.0	11.3	12.0	8.5	6.8	4.9	4.6	3.9	4.4	6.5	9.3	13.8
Firearm (E919)	100.0	8.9	6.0	6.3	6.9	6.0	6.2	7.1	7.6	7.8	11.4	14.1	11.7
Inhalation and ingestion causing obstruction or suffocation (E921, E922)	100.0	9.5	8.0	8.6	7.4	7.7	7.6	7.1	8.2	8.0	8.6	9.2	10.0
Drowning (E929)	100.0	2.9	3.0	4.5	6.8	11.7	17.2	21.2	15.3	7.7	4.0	2.9	2.9

Table 16   Death rates for motor-vehicle accidents, by age, color, and sex: United States, 1959-61 (E810-E835)

Age	Total			White			Nonwhite		
	Total	Male	Female	Total	Male	Female	Total	Male	Female
All ages	21.2	31.8	11.0	21.1	31.5	11.1	21.9	34.2	10.2
Under 1	7.8	7.8	7.8	8.0	8.0	8.1	6.4	6.8	6.1
1	10.0	10.8	9.3	10.2	10.8	9.6	9.2	10.7	7.7
2	9.2	10.4	8.0	9.0	10.2	7.7	10.4	11.1	9.8
3	9.7	11.5	7.9	9.5	11.3	7.8	10.9	13.0	8.8
4	10.0	11.9	8.0	9.6	11.3	7.9	12.1	15.3	8.9
5 - 14	7.8	10.4	5.2	7.7	10.2	5.1	8.7	11.5	5.8
15 - 24	37.7	61.2	14.7	38.8	62.8	15.2	29.9	49.2	11.8
25 - 34	24.4	40.0	9.5	23.7	38.5	9.3	29.9	51.4	11.4
35 - 44	19.4	30.2	9.2	18.6	28.6	9.0	27.0	44.4	11.3
45 - 54	21.5	31.8	11.5	20.7	30.1	11.4	29.7	47.7	12.6
55 - 64	24.8	35.5	14.8	24.3	34.2	14.9	30.8	48.3	13.8
65 - 74	31.6	45.9	19.1	31.6	45.7	19.4	31.2	48.8	15.1
75 - 84	42.0	65.5	23.9	42.8	66.6	24.5	32.2	51.4	15.1
85 & over	37.1	65.5	18.9	37.4	65.6	19.7	33.5	64.8	9.1*
Age-adjusted									
Total	22.5	34.6	11.0	22.3	34.0	11.0	24.4	39.3	10.8
Under 15	8.2	10.4	6.2	8.2	10.2	6.1	9.1	11.4	6.6
65 & over	34.4	51.6	20.3	34.7	51.8	20.7	31.5	50.1	14.9

Table 17   Death rates for all motor-vehicle accidents
and selected types of motor-vehicle accidents,
by age and sex: United States, 1959-61

Age and sex	Total motor-vehicle (E810-E835)	Total motor-vehicle traffic (E810-E825)	Pedestrian traffic (E812)	Involving two or more motor vehicles (E816)	Involving running off roadway (E823)
Both sexes	21.2	20.7	4.0	7.1	4.5
Under 5	9.3	7.8	3.6	2.1	0.7
5-14	7.8	7.6	3.6	1.3	0.6
15-24	37.7	37.3	1.8	11.5	12.2
25-34	24.4	24.0	1.6	8.7	7.0
35-44	19.4	19.1	2.1	7.4	4.9
45-54	21.5	21.0	3.4	8.6	4.3
55-64	24.8	24.3	6.1	10.0	3.6
65-74	31.6	30.9	10.9	11.7	3.4
75-84	42.0	41.2	19.3	13.0	3.4
85 & over	37.1	36.1	20.0	9.1	2.7
Males	31.8	30.9	5.9	9.7	7.3
Under 5	10.4	8.7	4.5	2.1	0.7
5-14	10.4	10.0	4.8	1.4	0.7
15-24	61.2	60.4	2.9	17.0	20.6
25-34	40.0	39.2	2.6	13.2	12.1
35-44	30.2	29.5	3.3	10.3	8.1
45-54	31.8	31.0	5.1	11.6	6.9
55-64	35.5	34.5	9.3	12.8	5.6
65-74	45.9	44.9	16.7	15.8	4.9
75-84	65.5	64.2	31.4	18.7	5.0
85 & over	65.5	63.9	39.8	13.4	4.1
Females	11.0	10.7	2.2	4.6	1.8
Under 5	8.2	6.8	2.7	2.2	0.7
5-14	5.2	5.1	2.3	1.3	0.5
15-24	14.7	14.7	0.7	6.0	4.0
25-34	9.5	9.4	0.7	4.3	2.0
35-44	9.2	9.2	0.9	4.5	1.8
45-54	11.5	11.4	1.6	5.8	1.8
55-64	14.8	14.6	3.1	7.4	1.7
65-74	19.1	18.8	5.9	8.1	2.0
75-84	23.9	23.4	9.8	8.6	2.1
85 & over	18.9	18.4	7.3	6.3	1.8

Table 18   Age-adjusted death rates for motor-vehicle accidents,
by color and sex: United States, each geographic division and state, 1959-61
(E810-E835)

Geographic area	Total			White			Nonwhite		
	Total	Male	Female	Total	Male	Female	Total	Male	Female
United States	22.5	34.6	11.0	22.3	34.0	11.0	24.4	39.3	10.8
New England	13.6	21.4	6.2	13.5	21.3	6.1	16.8	26.1	7.8
Connecticut	12.7	20.0	5.9	12.4	19.4	5.8	19.0	30.7	8.5*
Maine	18.4	29.0	7.7	18.3	28.8	7.7	50.0*	87.7*	-
Massachusetts	12.4	19.6	5.8	12.4	19.7	5.7	13.4	19.9	7.2*
New Hampshire	18.7	28.6	8.8	18.7	28.6	8.9	19.3*	33.9*	-
Rhode Island	9.2	14.2	4.2	9.0	13.9	4.0	18.7*	26.1*	11.2*
Vermont	23.9	38.5	9.9	24.0	38.6	9.9	-	-	-
Middle Atlantic	14.5	22.8	6.9	14.5	22.8	6.9	14.5	23.6	6.6
New Jersey	13.4	20.7	6.5	13.0	19.9	6.5	17.0	29.7	5.6
New York	13.9	21.8	6.7	13.9	21.8	6.7	14.0	22.3	6.9
Pennsylvania	16.0	25.5	7.3	16.2	25.8	7.4	14.0	22.1	6.7
East North Central	21.5	32.7	10.9	21.8	33.1	11.0	17.7	27.4	8.8
Illinois	18.1	27.8	9.0	18.5	28.2	9.2	15.1	23.9	7.2
Indiana	25.9	39.3	13.2	26.1	39.5	13.2	23.8	36.7	11.8
Michigan	22.8	34.1	12.0	23.3	34.8	12.3	16.8	25.6	8.5
Ohio	20.6	31.1	10.7	20.7	31.3	10.8	19.1	29.1	9.7
Wisconsin	24.5	38.3	11.2	24.5	38.4	11.2	25.9	39.1	12.8*
West North Central	25.4	38.8	12.6	25.2	38.4	12.4	31.8	48.6	16.1
Iowa	25.9	38.9	13.6	26.0	39.0	13.6	22.5*	28.9*	16.6*
Kansas	26.2	39.1	13.5	26.4	39.5	13.4	23.1	30.1	15.8
Minnesota	23.5	36.0	11.6	23.2	35.6	11.4	50.3	71.8	27.7*
Missouri	24.3	37.6	11.7	24.6	37.7	12.0	21.9	36.7	8.7
Nebraska	24.6	37.4	12.2	24.4	37.2	11.9	34.4	43.7	24.5*
North Dakota	28.8	42.4	14.6	27.5	41.4	13.2	100.1	109.0*	89.0*
South Dakota	37.2	58.1	16.0	32.0	50.2	13.5	166.3	257.4	75.7
South Atlantic	24.6	38.7	11.1	23.8	36.9	11.0	27.8	46.2	11.1
Delaware	18.8	31.6	6.6	17.5	29.9	5.8	27.8	42.9	12.5*
District of Columbia	12.4	20.3	5.4	11.5	18.1	5.3	12.7	22.0	4.7
Florida	25.2	37.9	12.8	24.1	35.9	12.6	30.9	48.7	13.9
Georgia	27.6	43.5	12.6	28.2	43.8	13.2	26.3	43.5	11.6
Maryland	17.4	26.9	8.3	16.3	25.1	7.8	23.6	37.2	10.4
North Carolina	29.9	48.5	12.1	28.9	45.6	12.3	34.3	59.3	11.4
South Carolina	30.5	48.2	13.7	30.3	46.2	14.4	31.8	54.4	12.3
Virginia	21.2	33.6	8.8	20.1	31.3	8.6	26.2	43.5	9.5
West Virginia	22.1	35.7	9.3	22.1	35.6	9.4	21.1	37.1	7.3*
East South Central	27.7	43.9	12.4	28.4	44.2	13.0	25.8	44.0	10.2
Alabama	30.7	49.2	13.7	31.9	49.7	15.0	28.3	49.1	10.8
Kentucky	26.5	42.4	10.7	26.6	42.4	10.9	25.2	43.5	8.0
Mississippi	30.1	48.3	13.3	33.5	51.6	15.7	25.6	44.5	9.9
Tennessee	24.7	38.3	12.0	25.2	38.8	12.3	22.6	36.4	10.6
West South Central	27.7	42.3	13.8	27.8	42.0	13.9	28.0	44.7	13.1
Arkansas	28.6	45.2	13.0	29.2	45.4	13.6	27.0	46.0	10.7
Louisiana	26.4	41.5	12.4	26.6	41.1	12.8	26.7	44.1	11.7
Oklahoma	30.8	45.1	16.9	29.9	43.7	16.3	41.1	61.9	22.4
Texas	27.3	41.5	13.6	27.4	41.5	13.7	26.9	42.0	13.3
Mountain	35.5	52.8	18.3	33.8	50.1	17.4	72.9	108.6	35.2
Arizona	36.7	54.9	18.4	33.1	49.4	16.8	72.9	111.0	33.2
Colorado	27.3	40.8	14.1	27.2	40.8	14.0	28.6	41.4	15.8*
Idaho	36.3	51.1	21.3	35.9	50.5	21.1	64.2*	83.5*	43.9*
Montana	40.4	61.0	19.3	38.1	58.0	17.7	117.3	159.0	71.5
Nevada	49.6	66.7	30.9	47.7	64.4	29.6	74.3	97.8	45.8*
New Mexico	43.4	67.6	18.8	39.9	61.8	17.6	91.6	146.2	35.9
Utah	29.5	41.1	18.4	28.3	39.2	18.0	93.6	139.4	42.4*
Wyoming	44.9	68.7	20.4	44.2	68.3	19.4	78.6*	94.7*	61.8*
Pacific	25.8	37.6	13.9	25.9	37.8	14.1	25.2	36.5	12.9
Alaska	18.0	22.9	10.6	17.7	22.1	10.9*	18.8	25.0*	10.8*
California	26.4	38.6	14.3	26.4	38.5	14.4	26.6	39.2	13.3
Hawaii	17.0	24.8	7.3	18.6	28.7	6.0*	16.0	23.1	7.9
Oregon	29.7	43.5	16.4	29.2	43.1	15.9	52.8	63.4	41.5*
Washington	23.1	33.8	12.4	22.6	33.0	12.1	39.2	55.5	19.7

Table 19   Death rates for motor-vehicle traffic accidents to pedestrians, by age, color, and sex: United States, 1959-61
(E812)

Age	Total			White			Nonwhite		
	Total	Male	Female	Total	Male	Female	Total	Male	Female
All ages	4.0	5.9	2.2	3.7	5.4	2.1	6.4	9.6	3.4
Under 1	0.2	0.3*	0.2*	0.2	0.3*	0.2*	0.3*	0.4*	0.2*
1	2.5	2.9	2.1	2.5	2.8	2.1	2.8	3.5	2.1*
2	4.0	5.1	3.0	3.8	4.8	2.7	5.7	6.5	4.9
3	5.3	6.8	3.7	4.9	6.3	3.4	7.7	9.6	5.8
4	6.1	7.6	4.4	5.5	6.9	4.0	9.5	12.3	6.8
5 - 14	3.6	4.8	2.3	3.3	4.5	2.1	5.2	6.9	3.6
15 - 24	1.8	2.9	0.7	1.6	2.6	0.7	3.4	5.6	1.3
25 - 34	1.6	2.6	0.7	1.2	2.0	0.5	4.6	7.6	2.0
35 - 44	2.1	3.3	0.9	1.7	2.6	0.7	5.5	9.0	2.4
45 - 54	3.4	5.1	1.6	2.9	4.3	1.5	7.8	12.7	3.1
55 - 64	6.1	9.3	3.1	5.5	8.4	2.8	12.3	18.3	6.5
65 - 74	10.9	16.7	5.9	10.4	15.9	5.7	16.6	25.9	8.2
75 - 84	19.3	31.4	9.8	19.2	31.4	9.9	20.3	32.5	9.3
85 & over	20.0	39.8	7.3	19.7	39.4	7.3	23.3	44.6	6.6*
Age-adjusted									
Total	3.6	5.4	1.9	3.2	4.9	1.7	6.6	10.1	3.3
Under 15	3.6	4.7	2.5	3.3	4.4	2.3	5.3	6.8	3.7
65 & over	13.4	21.3	6.9	13.0	20.8	6.8	17.8	28.3	8.4

Table 20   Age-adjusted death rates for motor-vehicle traffic accidents
to pedestrians, by color and sex: United States,
each geographic division and state, 1959-61
(E812)

Geographic area	Total			White			Nonwhite		
	Total	Male	Female	Total	Male	Female	Total	Male	Female
United States	3.6	5.4	1.9	3.2	4.9	1.7	6.6	10.1	3.3
New England	2.9	4.4	1.5	2.8	4.3	1.5	4.6	7.8	1.6*
Connecticut	2.4	3.4	1.5	2.3	3.3	1.5	3.6*	6.1*	1.3*
Maine	3.3	4.9	1.9	3.3	4.7	1.9	18.6*	31.4*	-
Massachusetts	3.2	5.1	1.6	3.2	5.0	1.6	5.4	8.6*	2.4*
New Hampshire	2.4	3.9	0.9*	2.4	3.9	0.9*	-	-	-
Rhode Island	2.0	3.2	0.9*	1.9	3.1	0.9*	4.5*	9.0*	-
Vermont	2.8	4.2	1.5*	2.8	4.2	1.5*	-	-	-
Middle Atlantic	3.6	5.4	2.0	3.4	5.1	1.8	5.7	8.2	3.3
New Jersey	3.5	5.2	2.0	3.4	4.9	1.9	5.1	8.6	1.8*
New York	3.7	5.6	2.1	3.5	5.3	1.9	6.2	9.2	3.7
Pennsylvania	3.4	5.2	1.8	3.3	5.0	1.7	5.0	6.5	3.5
East North Central	3.0	4.5	1.6	2.9	4.3	1.6	4.7	7.4	2.2
Illinois	2.8	4.3	1.4	2.6	4.0	1.4	4.3	6.9	1.8
Indiana	2.6	3.9	1.4	2.5	3.7	1.3	5.5	8.4	2.8*
Michigan	3.5	5.3	1.8	3.4	5.2	1.8	4.2	7.2	1.4*
Ohio	3.1	4.6	1.8	2.9	4.3	1.8	5.4	7.8	3.0
Wisconsin	2.9	4.3	1.6	2.8	4.2	1.5	7.2*	10.5*	3.8*
West North Central	2.5	3.8	1.4	2.3	3.4	1.3	8.0	13.3	2.9
Iowa	1.9	2.7	1.3	1.9	2.6	1.3	5.3*	9.1*	1.8*
Kansas	1.8	2.5	1.0	1.7	2.5	0.9	3.5*	5.0*	2.2*
Minnesota	3.0	4.4	1.6	2.9	4.2	1.6	12.3*	18.1*	6.2*
Missouri	3.1	4.8	1.5	2.8	4.2	1.5	6.6	11.4	2.2*
Nebraska	1.9	2.6	1.3	1.8	2.4	1.2	9.7*	9.9*	9.5*
North Dakota	1.7	2.8	0.5*	1.5	2.4	0.5*	14.7*	28.1*	-
South Dakota	3.3	5.4	1.2*	1.9	3.0	0.8*	38.5	68.7	8.4*
South Atlantic	4.4	6.7	2.3	3.5	5.3	1.9	8.0	12.4	4.0
Delaware	2.3	3.3	1.4*	2.0	3.0*	1.2*	4.6*	5.4*	3.8*
District of Columbia	4.6	8.1	1.6	3.3	5.1	1.8*	5.5	10.5	1.1*
Florida	4.4	6.6	2.4	3.7	5.5	1.9	8.7	13.1	4.5
Georgia	4.2	6.3	2.4	3.6	5.4	2.0	6.1	8.8	3.8
Maryland	4.3	6.6	2.3	3.5	5.4	2.0	8.6	13.2	3.9
North Carolina	5.2	8.0	2.6	4.0	6.1	2.1	9.2	14.5	4.5
South Carolina	5.6	8.5	3.0	3.9	5.8	2.1	9.7	15.4	4.9
Virginia	4.0	6.2	1.9	3.1	4.7	1.5	8.0	12.4	3.7
West Virginia	3.1	4.8	1.5	2.9	4.5	1.4	6.9	9.9*	3.7*
East South Central	4.2	6.5	2.0	3.7	5.8	1.8	6.0	9.5	2.9
Alabama	4.7	7.2	2.4	3.8	5.7	2.0	7.1	11.3	3.5
Kentucky	3.9	6.2	1.8	3.9	6.1	1.8	4.8	7.7	1.9*
Mississippi	4.4	7.0	1.9	3.7	5.9	1.7	5.4	9.0	2.4
Tennessee	3.8	6.0	1.9	3.5	5.5	1.6	5.5	8.6	2.9
West South Central	3.6	5.5	1.8	3.1	4.8	1.5	6.1	9.3	3.2
Arkansas	3.3	4.9	1.7	2.8	4.3	1.4	5.1	7.8	2.8
Louisiana	4.7	7.4	2.2	3.8	6.4	1.4	6.8	10.2	3.8
Oklahoma	2.8	4.0	1.7	2.5	3.3	1.6	6.7	11.5	2.5*
Texas	3.5	5.4	1.7	3.1	5.0	1.5	5.8	8.9	2.9
Mountain	4.2	6.4	2.1	3.5	5.3	1.8	19.8	30.0	8.6
Arizona	6.6	10.2	3.1	5.0	7.9	2.2	23.9	34.8	12.1*
Colorado	2.7	4.1	1.4	2.6	4.0	1.3	5.6*	8.1*	3.1*
Idaho	3.3	5.4	1.1*	3.0	4.8	1.1*	24.1*	44.6*	-
Montana	2.4	3.3	1.6*	2.2	2.8	1.5*	13.9*	22.7*	3.0*
Nevada	5.4	6.5	4.2*	4.7	5.8	3.5*	14.8*	16.8*	12.8*
New Mexico	6.0	9.6	2.3	4.7	7.6	1.8	24.7	37.9	10.9*
Utah	4.4	6.8	2.1	4.0	6.0	2.0	31.7*	53.4*	4.8*
Wyoming	3.1	4.0	2.2*	2.8	3.3*	2.3*	24.9*	45.6*	-
Pacific	4.0	6.0	2.2	3.8	5.7	2.1	6.2	8.8	3.4
Alaska	3.5*	5.0*	1.1*	1.6*	2.3*	0.6*	10.0*	15.2*	3.2*
California	4.2	6.3	2.4	4.1	6.0	2.3	6.4	8.7	3.9
Hawaii	4.9	7.1	2.2*	4.5*	7.9*	1.2*	5.1	7.1	2.7*
Oregon	3.4	5.3	1.7	3.3	5.1	1.6	7.9*	13.5*	2.5*
Washington	3.3	4.8	1.9	3.2	4.5	1.9	6.7*	12.1*	-

Table 21　　　Age-adjusted death rates for motor-vehicle traffic accidents
to pedestrians under age 15, by color and sex: United States,
each geographic division and state, 1959-61
(E812)

Geographic area	Total			White			Nonwhite		
	Total	Male	Female	Total	Male	Female	Total	Male	Female
United States	3.6	4.7	2.5	3.3	4.4	2.3	5.3	6.8	3.7
New England	3.3	4.5	2.1	3.4	4.5	2.0	2.8*	3.1*	2.5*
Connecticut	2.3	2.8	1.6*	2.4	2.9	1.8*	1.6*	2.0*	1.2*
Maine	5.3	6.9	3.7*	5.4	6.9	3.7*	-	-	-
Massachusetts	3.5	4.9	2.1	3.5	4.9	2.0	4.5*	4.8*	4.2*
New Hampshire	3.5*	4.9*	1.9*	3.5*	4.9*	1.9*	-	-	-
Rhode Island	2.4*	3.5*	1.3*	2.5*	3.6*	1.3*	-	-	-
Vermont	3.6*	5.4*	1.8*	3.6*	5.4*	1.8*	-	-	-
Middle Atlantic	3.5	4.6	2.4	3.4	4.4	2.2	5.0	6.7	3.3
New Jersey	3.1	4.0	2.2	3.0	3.8	2.1	4.2	6.0*	2.6*
New York	3.3	4.3	2.3	3.1	4.1	2.2	4.4	6.2	2.8*
Pennsylvania	3.9	5.4	2.6	3.7	5.0	2.4	6.3	8.1	4.5
East North Central	3.3	4.4	2.1	3.1	4.1	2.0	4.9	7.0	3.0
Illinois	2.6	3.5	1.6	2.3	2.9	1.5	5.1	7.3	2.9*
Indiana	2.9	3.8	1.9	2.8	3.9	1.6	3.8*	2.9*	4.8*
Michigan	4.0	5.5	2.4	3.9	5.4	2.5	4.1	6.9	1.4*
Ohio	3.5	4.7	2.4	3.4	4.4	2.4	5.7	7.5	3.7*
Wisconsin	3.0	4.1	1.9	2.9	3.9	1.8	7.9*	11.3*	4.5*
West North Central	2.7	3.4	1.9	2.6	3.2	1.9	5.1	7.8	2.7*
Iowa	2.4	2.2	2.5	2.4	2.2	2.5	3.6*	-	7.1*
Kansas	2.5	3.6	1.3*	2.5	3.6	1.2*	4.1*	6.0*	2.3*
Minnesota	2.8	3.9	1.6	2.8	3.8	1.8	3.3*	6.3*	-
Missouri	3.0	3.9	2.1	2.7	3.4	2.1	5.3	8.2*	2.4*
Nebraska	2.5	3.2	1.8*	2.4	2.9*	1.9*	4.6*	9.2*	-
North Dakota	1.6*	3.0*	0.3*	1.4*	2.5*	0.3*	10.1*	19.7*	-
South Dakota	3.1	4.0*	2.1*	2.7*	3.7*	1.5*	10.5*	9.6*	11.1*
South Atlantic	4.9	6.3	3.4	4.3	5.7	3.0	6.3	8.1	4.6
Delaware	1.8*	2.2*	1.3*	1.9*	2.1*	1.5*	1.1*	2.4*	-
District of Columbia	5.3	8.9	1.6*	2.7*	4.2*	1.1*	6.3	10.7	1.9*
Florida	4.5	6.3	2.8	4.0	5.9	2.1	6.4	7.4	5.3
Georgia	4.8	6.3	3.3	4.7	6.0	3.3	5.1	6.9	3.4
Maryland	4.4	5.7	3.2	4.0	4.9	3.2	6.0	8.6	3.4*
North Carolina	6.4	7.3	5.4	5.5	6.3	4.6	8.1	9.5	6.9
South Carolina	6.7	8.2	4.8	6.0	7.7	4.1	7.5	9.1	6.0
Virginia	3.6	5.1	2.1	3.4	4.7	2.0	4.4	6.4	2.5*
West Virginia	3.7	5.3	2.2*	3.7	5.3	2.1*	5.1*	6.2*	4.1*
East South Central	4.4	5.7	3.0	4.2	5.4	3.1	4.8	6.6	3.1
Alabama	5.1	6.2	4.0	4.9	5.6	4.3	5.5	7.3	3.7
Kentucky	4.2	6.0	2.6	4.4	6.1	2.8	2.6*	4.3*	0.8*
Mississippi	4.2	5.3	3.0	3.5	3.7	3.2*	4.8	6.9	2.7*
Tennessee	3.9	5.1	2.6	3.8	5.1	2.4	4.3	5.4*	3.3*
West South Central	3.3	4.2	2.3	3.1	4.1	2.0	4.2	4.6	3.8
Arkansas	3.6	4.5	2.6	3.3	4.3	2.2*	4.5	5.1*	3.9*
Louisiana	3.8	5.0	2.7	3.2	4.7	1.5*	4.9	5.7	4.4
Oklahoma	2.8	3.3	2.2	3.0	3.6	2.4	1.3*	0.9*	1.8*
Texas	3.2	4.1	2.2	3.1	4.1	2.0	3.8	4.1	3.6
Mountain	3.5	4.6	2.4	3.4	4.6	2.3	4.8	4.5*	5.3*
Arizona	3.8	5.0	2.6*	4.0	5.5	2.5*	2.9*	2.3*	3.6*
Colorado	2.7	3.7	1.6*	2.5	3.7	1.3*	8.2*	4.1*	12.6*
Idaho	3.8	5.1*	2.4*	3.7	4.9*	2.4*	9.3*	19.1*	-
Montana	2.2*	2.4*	2.1*	2.1*	2.5*	1.5*	6.0*	-	12.1*
Nevada	6.0*	5.5*	6.5*	5.3*	4.2*	6.5*	12.7*	19.6*	5.9*
New Mexico	3.4	4.8	2.0*	3.6	4.9	2.2*	2.0*	3.9*	-
Utah	4.9	7.0	2.9*	4.8	6.9	2.6*	15.1*	11.3*	19.0*
Wyoming	3.0*	3.0*	3.1*	3.1*	3.0*	3.2*	-	-	-
Pacific	3.2	4.2	2.2	3.1	4.1	2.1	4.7	6.1	3.4
Alaska	2.8*	3.2*	2.4*	2.5*	2.7*	2.4*	3.4*	4.4*	2.4*
California	3.4	4.5	2.3	3.2	4.3	2.1	5.6	6.5	4.6
Hawaii	2.9*	4.0*	1.9*	1.2*	-	2.5*	3.6*	5.6*	1.6*
Oregon	2.9	3.5	2.3*	2.9	3.3	2.3*	5.5*	11.0*	-
Washington	2.7	3.6	1.6	2.8	3.7	1.8	0.7*	1.4*	-

Table 22   Age-adjusted death rates for motor-vehicle traffic accidents
to pedestrians age 65 and over, by color and sex: United States,
each geographic division and state, 1959-61
(E812)

Geographic area	Total			White			Nonwhite		
	Total	Male	Female	Total	Male	Female	Total	Male	Female
United States	13.4	21.3	6.9	13.0	20.8	6.8	17.8	28.3	8.4
New England	12.9	20.8	7.2	12.8	20.3	7.2	25.4*	48.1*	4.7*
Connecticut	12.7	18.7	8.3	12.3	17.8	8.1	37.6*	65.0*	14.1*
Maine	12.1	18.6	6.8*	12.1	18.6	6.8*	-	-	-
Massachusetts	14.3	23.6	7.7	14.2	23.2	7.8	23.9*	50.1*	-
New Hampshire	9.5	18.4*	2.8*	9.5	18.5*	2.8*	-	-	-
Rhode Island	9.6	15.2*	5.8*	9.7	15.4*	5.9*	-	-	-
Vermont	10.6*	18.3*	4.8*	10.6*	18.3*	4.8*	-	-	-
Middle Atlantic	15.3	24.8	8.0	15.3	24.8	7.9	16.5	25.1	9.1
New Jersey	14.4	22.8	8.1	14.6	22.7	8.5	11.3*	24.2*	-
New York	16.9	27.2	9.1	16.8	27.0	9.0	18.8	30.4	9.5*
Pennsylvania	13.5	22.4	6.2	13.4	22.6	6.0	16.1	19.0*	12.9*
East North Central	12.8	20.6	6.5	12.7	20.4	6.4	15.8	25.5	6.9*
Illinois	12.7	20.2	6.6	12.5	20.2	6.3	14.7	19.1*	11.0*
Indiana	11.1	17.3	6.0	10.4	16.0	6.0	28.3*	50.2*	6.8*
Michigan	15.5	26.0	6.4	15.5	25.9	6.7	14.3*	29.7*	-
Ohio	12.5	19.2	7.1	12.5	19.2	7.0	12.4*	18.1*	7.3*
Wisconsin	12.4	20.0	5.8	12.2	19.6	5.8	33.1*	63.2*	-
West North Central	8.7	13.8	4.5	8.5	13.2	4.5	18.8	32.8	5.5*
Iowa	5.9	9.4	3.1*	6.0	9.5	3.2*	-	-	-
Kansas	5.7	8.5	3.3*	5.6	8.3	3.5*	7.7*	15.6*	-
Minnesota	11.7	17.5	6.6	11.5	17.2	6.4	41.0*	52.1*	30.4*
Missouri	11.5	19.6	4.9	10.9	18.2	5.0	20.6	38.8*	4.1*
Nebraska	6.9	9.7	4.5*	6.7	9.9	4.1*	15.1*	-	31.0*
North Dakota	5.9*	7.5*	4.2*	5.3*	6.3*	4.3*	70.3*	136.2*	-
South Dakota	5.4*	9.0*	1.8*	5.0*	8.2*	1.9*	25.0*	44.9*	-
South Atlantic	12.3	20.0	6.0	11.1	18.1	5.6	17.9	29.4	8.3
Delaware	11.6*	20.3*	4.7*	11.0*	20.7*	3.6*	17.7*	17.5*	17.9*
District of Columbia	14.0	21.8*	9.1*	13.3*	16.4*	11.3*	15.6*	32.9*	3.0*
Florida	12.3	18.0	6.8	11.3	16.1	6.7	23.9	41.0	8.5*
Georgia	12.6	22.4	5.5	12.6	22.2	5.7	12.9	23.3	5.2*
Maryland	14.5	26.3	6.2	13.7	24.7	6.1	21.0*	35.7*	7.0*
North Carolina	14.0	25.1	5.3	12.4	23.0	4.2*	20.4	32.7	9.9*
South Carolina	10.5	18.2	4.8*	9.0	17.0	3.2*	14.0	21.2*	8.5*
Virginia	10.6	16.0	6.5	8.3	13.0	4.9	20.1	26.9	13.9*
West Virginia	9.4	14.1	4.9*	9.0	13.2	5.1*	14.9*	27.0*	-
East South Central	13.2	22.0	5.8	12.9	22.0	5.4	14.1	21.7	7.4
Alabama	13.7	23.0	6.1	12.2	22.2	4.2*	17.0	24.6	10.9*
Kentucky	14.5	23.0	7.2	14.9	23.8	7.3	10.0*	14.4*	6.2*
Mississippi	13.0	21.3	5.9*	12.4	21.3	5.2*	13.9	21.3	7.1*
Tennessee	11.7	20.6	4.3	11.6	20.4	4.5	11.5*	21.0*	2.8*
West South Central	11.1	18.0	5.4	10.0	16.3	4.9	17.0	26.9	8.0
Arkansas	10.0	15.1	5.2*	8.7	13.3	4.3*	15.0*	21.6*	8.7*
Louisiana	14.0	22.5	7.3	12.8	21.8	6.0*	16.4	23.9	10.0*
Oklahoma	9.3	12.7	6.4	8.3	11.4	5.7	20.3*	26.4*	14.4*
Texas	11.0	19.2	4.5	10.2	17.5	4.4	17.6	31.8	4.5*
Mountain	14.7	23.1	7.0	14.1	21.6	7.1	36.6*	66.0*	-
Arizona	27.2	44.0	11.1*	26.5	42.5	11.7*	36.7*	63.9*	-
Colorado	9.5	14.2	5.6*	9.5	14.0	5.7*	9.3*	19.3*	-
Idaho	13.5	23.6	3.7*	13.0	22.7	3.7*	54.6*	100.7*	-
Montana	7.4*	8.9*	5.8*	6.6*	7.1*	5.9*	53.9*	97.5*	-
Nevada	19.9*	24.2*	15.8*	18.9*	21.7*	16.7*	40.2*	75.8*	-
New Mexico	16.7	29.6	4.0*	16.2	28.8	4.2*	24.8*	43.0*	-
Utah	15.4	25.5	7.0*	14.5	23.6	7.0*	73.0*	113.4*	-
Wyoming	16.4*	22.0*	10.5*	14.2*	17.6*	10.6*	165.6*	286.4*	-
Pacific	18.1	27.4	10.7	17.6	26.7	10.3	29.8	39.0	19.4
Alaska	12.6*	20.4*	-	-	-	-	45.5*	80.0*	-
California	18.9	28.8	11.4	18.6	28.5	11.1	27.4	34.6	20.0*
Hawaii	32.8	46.4	17.0*	23.0*	50.1*	-	36.0	45.0*	24.2*
Oregon	13.1	21.2	5.8*	13.1	21.1	5.9*	18.0*	31.9*	-
Washington	15.9	23.3	9.3	15.7	22.7	9.4	30.5*	55.2*	-

160

Table 23   Death rates for motor-vehicle accidents, excluding pedestrian traffic,
by age: United States, each geographic division and state, 1959-61
(E810, E811, E813-E835)

Geographic area	All ages	Under 5	5-14	15-24	25-34	35-44	45-54	55-64	65-74	75-84	85 & over
United States	17.2	5.7	4.2	35.9	22.8	17.3	18.1	18.7	20.7	22.7	17.1
New England	9.5	3.0	2.3	25.8	12.0	8.3	7.8	8.6	9.4	11.6	8.5
Connecticut	8.9	2.1	2.4	25.7	11.9	8.8	6.6	7.7	7.0	10.7	7.1*
Maine	13.4	5.2	3.3	35.8	17.2	11.5	11.6	10.3	14.6	12.2	17.2*
Massachusetts	8.2	2.4	1.7	22.1	9.8	7.0	6.7	8.3	9.2	11.7	6.6
New Hampshire	14.1	4.6*	4.2	40.9	21.6	11.4	8.7	9.3	12.4	16.7*	14.0*
Rhode Island	6.5	2.3*	1.3*	17.6	8.6	4.8	6.2	6.1	5.0	5.3*	13.0*
Vermont	19.1	9.1*	5.1	40.6	23.5	20.6	22.4	19.8	18.6	19.6*	0.0*
Middle Atlantic	9.8	2.3	2.1	23.7	12.9	9.0	9.7	10.0	11.4	12.9	9.3
New Jersey	8.9	2.0	1.8	21.7	11.4	7.3	8.9	10.2	10.1	13.8	11.9
New York	9.1	2.0	2.1	22.3	12.2	8.2	8.8	8.6	10.0	12.2	9.2
Pennsylvania	11.3	2.9	2.3	26.6	14.7	11.2	11.2	12.3	14.1	13.4	8.2
East North Central	16.7	5.1	4.3	35.3	21.2	15.9	17.3	20.3	22.3	25.0	18.1
Illinois	14.0	4.1	3.8	28.8	18.1	13.1	14.9	16.7	17.8	20.2	19.3
Indiana	21.3	6.8	6.0	42.7	25.6	21.4	23.8	26.3	27.5	30.0	20.7
Michigan	17.3	5.6	3.9	35.8	21.5	17.8	17.9	21.7	25.4	30.5	20.3
Ohio	15.8	4.8	4.2	31.8	21.6	14.8	16.2	20.1	21.4	22.8	15.2
Wisconsin	19.0	5.1	4.2	49.9	22.3	16.4	18.0	21.7	24.5	27.1	16.2
West North Central	21.1	7.4	5.5	43.6	25.4	20.4	22.8	23.5	28.2	30.0	20.3
Iowa	22.2	7.2	6.7	45.3	24.5	22.1	25.3	24.8	29.5	31.4	20.8
Kansas	23.0	9.5	7.1	45.2	25.6	22.9	22.3	24.8	33.9	34.2	42.5
Minnesota	18.6	6.4	4.5	39.7	20.5	19.1	21.1	22.3	26.1	27.7	12.7*
Missouri	19.5	7.3	4.2	40.9	25.7	18.1	22.0	19.9	22.6	26.2	17.6
Nebraska	20.9	8.5	4.6	46.2	23.2	18.7	21.0	24.2	31.4	28.2	6.4*
North Dakota	24.3	6.3	8.2	44.8	33.6	28.4	24.4	30.9	32.6	38.2	10.0*
South Dakota	30.1	6.8	7.3	63.2	48.4	23.3	30.3	37.2	43.2	44.2	33.0*
South Atlantic	18.4	5.6	4.7	37.3	25.7	20.5	19.1	19.5	18.8	21.2	17.8
Delaware	14.5	2.4	2.3	33.2	23.0	13.5	11.6	15.5	28.4	13.2	15.9*
District of Columbia	7.4	1.7*	2.0	14.4	10.1	10.4	7.3	6.2	4.3	3.6	0.0*
Florida	19.2	7.4	5.8	35.8	24.6	21.4	21.3	19.8	21.3	27.9	27.7
Georgia	21.0	6.4	5.3	41.1	31.0	24.0	24.9	22.2	21.3	18.8	19.0*
Maryland	11.8	2.9	3.1	24.3	15.5	13.0	11.9	14.7	13.4	17.3	16.0*
North Carolina	22.5	7.0	5.2	47.5	32.0	25.6	22.5	24.2	20.1	19.2	12.2*
South Carolina	22.3	8.5	6.3	37.9	37.1	27.6	24.3	23.1	23.6	27.7	17.9*
Virginia	15.7	3.7	3.7	34.3	21.6	16.2	16.1	16.6	13.8	21.4	14.0*
West Virginia	16.8	3.1	3.3	40.7	21.9	19.7	13.7	19.5	19.1	18.2	16.8*
East South Central	21.2	7.8	4.6	41.3	30.9	23.2	26.5	21.4	23.0	21.5	20.0
Alabama	23.5	9.4	5.9	41.3	34.7	26.2	30.2	26.5	28.2	22.3	32.8*
Kentucky	20.0	5.1	3.3	45.7	28.9	20.0	24.9	18.5	21.4	18.5	15.1*
Mississippi	22.6	9.1	4.3	39.4	36.2	29.6	29.8	24.6	24.1	26.6	20.2*
Tennessee	19.2	7.5	4.7	38.7	26.3	19.7	22.6	17.9	19.4	20.7	14.9*
West South Central	22.1	8.3	6.1	39.2	29.2	24.8	25.7	27.2	28.4	30.5	21.6
Arkansas	23.2	7.9	6.4	44.2	30.6	26.0	26.2	25.2	27.4	30.5	24.1*
Louisiana	19.3	6.7	5.0	36.2	29.2	20.8	22.4	25.0	21.9	23.1	14.3*
Oklahoma	26.3	9.3	7.7	47.3	31.0	27.7	30.7	32.3	33.1	31.6	22.1
Texas	21.9	8.6	6.0	37.3	28.5	25.2	25.4	27.0	29.4	32.6	23.1
Mountain	28.0	10.0	6.7	55.8	37.2	29.2	33.1	32.9	36.9	41.5	35.5
Arizona	26.7	10.2	4.0	53.1	37.3	29.8	31.2	32.7	33.0	38.5	40.8*
Colorado	22.5	6.9	7.0	41.3	28.6	23.7	26.6	27.4	30.1	27.5	32.6*
Idaho	29.9	13.0	8.5	51.2	38.9	32.3	40.6	32.6	48.6	38.6	10.3*
Montana	33.7	8.0	7.6	73.1	47.6	31.4	38.7	36.6	40.3	66.3	30.0*
Nevada	41.3	11.1	8.6	69.6	43.9	44.6	60.6	61.7	55.4	63.4*	0.0*
New Mexico	33.0	14.4	7.2	71.0	48.6	35.0	32.4	38.1	34.3	37.1	58.9*
Utah	22.4	8.5	6.6	44.9	27.2	19.4	27.7	23.8	38.1	53.9	30.8*
Wyoming	36.7	12.3	7.1	92.1	45.8	36.0	32.4	40.6	45.5	47.5*	101.1*
Pacific	20.0	7.3	4.4	39.5	27.3	20.7	21.3	21.7	25.2	26.5	19.5
Alaska	13.0	3.9	2.9	23.8	16.0*	17.7	15.8	3.6*	35.6*	24.6*	-
California	20.3	7.5	4.3	40.3	28.3	20.7	21.5	21.8	25.1	26.8	17.0
Hawaii	11.1	4.1	2.5	26.0	11.8	11.1	13.4	10.5	10.2	8.4*	21.1*
Oregon	24.0	7.9	6.5	47.2	30.5	25.6	27.6	27.0	30.7	27.7	26.5*
Washington	18.2	6.5	3.9	35.6	24.7	20.2	17.5	20.3	23.8	26.4	27.3

Table 24   Death **rates** for motor-vehicle accidents, excluding pedestrian traffic,
by age, color, and sex: United States, 1959-61
(E810, E811, E813-E835)

Age	Total			White			Nonwhite		
	Total	Male	Female	Total	Male	Female	Total	Male	Female
All ages	17.2	25.9	8.8	17.4	26.1	9.0	15.5	24.6	6.8
Under 1	7.6	7.5	7.6	7.8	7.7	7.9	6.1	6.4	5.9
1	7.5	7.9	7.2	7.7	8.0	7.5	6.4	7.2	5.6
2	5.2	5.3	5.0	5.2	5.4	5.0	4.7	4.6	4.9
3	4.4	4.7	4.2	4.6	5.0	4.4	3.2	3.4	3.0
4	3.9	4.3	3.6	4.1	4.4	3.9	2.6	3.0	2.1*
5 - 14	4.2	5.6	2.9	4.4	5.7	3.0	3.5	4.6	2.2
15 - 24	35.9	58.3	14.0	37.2	60.2	14.5	26.5	43.6	10.5
25 - 34	22.8	37.4	8.8	22.5	36.5	8.8	25.3	43.8	9.4
35 - 44	17.3	26.9	8.3	16.9	26.0	8.3	21.5	35.4	8.9
45 - 54	18.1	26.7	9.9	17.8	25.8	9.9	21.9	35.0	9.5
55 - 64	18.7	26.2	11.7	18.8	25.8	12.1	18.5	30.0	7.3
65 - 74	20.7	29.2	13.2	21.2	29.8	13.7	14.6	22.9	6.9
75 - 84	22.7	34.1	14.1	23.6	35.2	14.6	11.9	18.9	5.8
85 & over	17.1	25.7	11.6	17.7	26.2	12.4	10.2	20.2	2.5*

Table 25   Death rates for motor-vehicle accidents, excluding pedestrian traffic,
persons age 15 and over, by color, sex,
and marital status: United States, 1959-61
(E810, E811, E813-E835)

Age and sex	White					Nonwhite				
	Total	Single	Married	Widowed	Divorced	Total	Single	Married	Widowed	Divorced
Male	35.2	54.0	26.6	49.7	89.6	37.0	42.2	32.5	37.9	61.7
15 - 19	50.2	49.4	56.1	156.3*	128.3*	31.1	30.1	42.6	132.3*	-
20 - 24	72.1	91.6	45.8	275.1	184.2	59.3	67.1	45.1	131.6*	86.4
25 - 29	42.3	61.0	34.1	220.2	161.2	49.9	59.3	42.9	116.0*	107.7
30 - 34	31.4	42.9	27.1	129.6	120.5	38.3	47.8	33.8	68.0*	67.3
35 - 39	26.2	33.6	22.8	103.5	103.6	36.9	44.0	32.3	54.9*	78.2
40 - 44	25.6	32.5	22.6	71.3	90.4	34.3	37.9	30.6	75.1	59.1
45 - 49	26.0	29.7	23.1	64.8	82.4	36.8	41.2	32.8	68.9	58.4
50 - 54	25.3	25.0	22.7	60.7	67.5	33.3	30.4	30.2	50.8	48.6
55 - 59	24.9	22.7	22.7	53.5	53.2	28.7	23.0	27.1	33.1	53.2
60 - 64	26.8	24.6	24.1	49.7	58.5	31.2	26.6*	27.4	44.6	58.1*
65 - 69	29.1	25.1	25.8	50.2	57.8	26.2	13.4*	25.2	33.0	37.9*
70 - 74	32.0	24.9	27.9	48.1	60.0	18.3	18.7*	16.2	22.6	-
75 - 79	36.5	31.7	31.9	45.9	64.3	19.7	5.2*	22.1	14.8*	46.0*
80 - 84	36.8	25.4	36.1	39.3	34.3*	18.3	12.9*	15.6*	21.8*	-
85 & over	28.4	15.1*	30.6	28.9	23.5*	22.1*	-	27.0*	18.6*	-
Female	11.1	12.8	9.6	14.0	21.6	9.0	10.0	8.3	8.9	13.1
15 - 19	15.6	15.2	15.5	122.7*	65.4	9.8	9.6	8.8	27.3*	34.8*
20 - 24	13.2	17.2	10.5	65.6	46.7	11.4	14.0	9.1	32.9*	25.1*
25 - 29	9.4	10.8	8.1	52.8	41.0	10.1	14.1	8.8	29.5*	10.7*
30 - 34	8.1	8.4	7.1	39.7	27.1	8.6	7.1*	7.5	22.4*	17.1*
35 - 39	8.1	6.7	7.1	31.2	23.5	8.3	7.5*	7.6	12.6*	15.3*
40 - 44	8.4	5.3	7.7	18.3	21.1	9.6	8.4*	8.4	16.0	13.8*
45 - 49	9.4	5.9	8.9	16.1	15.9	8.9	6.0*	8.2	12.5	12.3*
50 - 54	10.4	4.4	10.1	15.4	14.2	10.0	5.8*	10.1	9.7	10.9*
55 - 59	11.3	7.1	11.3	13.0	12.2	7.1	3.4*	7.0	8.6	3.6*
60 - 64	12.9	8.5	13.6	12.4	13.5	7.2	4.6*	7.5	6.8	9.8*
65 - 69	13.5	9.0	15.0	12.7	8.9	7.0	2.8*	8.1	6.1	9.6*
70 - 74	14.3	10.0	17.6	12.2	14.3	6.7	-	7.9*	6.8	-
75 - 79	15.2	11.6	20.7	13.1	14.1*	5.6*	6.6*	5.1*	5.3*	20.9*
80 - 84	14.8	9.0	21.9	13.8	21.0*	6.2*	14.0*	12.7*	4.8*	-
85 & over	13.2	8.1*	18.4	13.2	8.3*	2.6*	-	-	3.1*	-

Table 26   Age-adjusted death rates for motor-vehicle accidents,
excluding pedestrian traffic, by color and sex: United States,
each geographic division and state, 1959-61
(E810, E811, E813-E835)

Geographic area	Total			White			Nonwhite		
	Total	Male	Female	Total	Male	Female	Total	Male	Female
United States	18.9	29.2	9.1	19.1	29.1	9.3	17.8	29.2	7.5
New England	10.7	17.0	4.7	10.7	17.0	4.6	12.2	18.3	6.2
Connecticut	10.3	16.6	4.4	10.1	16.1	4.3	15.4	24.6	7.2*
Maine	15.1	24.1	5.8	15.0	24.1	5.8	31.4*	56.3*	-
Massachusetts	9.2	14.5	4.2	9.2	14.7	4.1	8.0	11.3*	4.8*
New Hampshire	16.3	24.7	7.9	16.3	24.7	8.0	19.3*	33.9*	-
Rhode Island	7.2	11.0	3.3	7.1	10.8	3.1	14.2*	17.1*	11.2*
Vermont	21.1	34.3	8.4	21.2	34.4	8.4	-	-	-
Middle Atlantic	10.9	17.4	4.9	11.1	17.7	5.1	8.8	15.4	3.3
New Jersey	9.9	15.5	4.5	9.6	15.0	4.6	11.9	21.1	3.8
New York	10.2	16.2	4.6	10.4	16.5	4.8	7.8	13.1	3.2
Pennsylvania	12.6	20.3	5.5	12.9	20.8	5.7	9.0	15.6	3.2
East North Central	18.5	28.2	9.3	18.9	28.8	9.4	13.0	20.0	6.6
Illinois	15.3	23.5	7.6	15.9	24.2	7.8	10.8	17.0	5.4
Indiana	23.3	35.4	11.8	23.6	35.8	11.9	18.3	28.3	9.0
Michigan	19.3	28.8	10.2	19.9	29.6	10.5	12.6	18.4	7.1
Ohio	17.5	26.5	8.9	17.8	27.0	9.0	13.7	21.3	6.7
Wisconsin	21.6	34.0	9.6	21.7	34.2	9.7	18.7	28.6	9.0*
West North Central	22.9	35.0	11.2	22.9	35.0	11.1	23.8	35.3	13.2
Iowa	24.0	36.2	12.3	24.1	36.4	12.3	17.2	19.8*	14.8*
Kansas	24.4	36.6	12.5	24.7	37.0	12.5	19.6	25.1	13.6
Minnesota	20.5	31.6	10.0	20.3	31.4	9.8	38.0	53.7	21.5*
Missouri	21.2	32.8	10.2	21.8	33.5	10.5	15.3	25.3	6.5
Nebraska	22.7	34.8	10.9	22.6	34.8	10.7	24.7	33.8	15.0*
North Dakota	27.1	39.6	14.1	26.0	39.0	12.7	85.4	80.9*	89.0*
South Dakota	33.9	52.7	14.8	30.1	47.2	12.7	127.8	188.7	67.3
South Atlantic	20.2	32.0	8.8	20.3	31.6	9.1	19.8	33.8	7.1
Delaware	16.5	28.3	5.2	15.5	26.9	4.6	23.2	37.5	8.7*
District of Columbia	7.8	12.2	3.8	8.2	13.0	3.5	7.2	11.5	3.6
Florida	20.8	31.3	10.4	20.4	30.4	10.7	22.2	35.6	9.4
Georgia	23.4	37.2	10.2	24.6	38.4	11.2	20.2	34.7	7.8
Maryland	13.1	20.3	6.0	12.8	19.7	5.8	15.0	24.0	6.5
North Carolina	24.7	40.5	9.5	24.9	39.5	10.2	25.1	44.8	6.9
South Carolina	24.9	39.7	10.7	26.4	40.4	12.3	22.1	39.0	7.4
Virginia	17.2	27.4	6.9	17.0	26.6	7.1	18.2	31.1	5.8
West Virginia	19.0	30.9	7.8	19.2	31.1	8.0	14.2	27.2	3.6*
East South Central	23.5	37.4	10.4	24.7	38.4	11.2	19.8	34.5	7.3
Alabama	26.0	42.0	11.3	28.1	44.0	13.0	21.2	37.8	7.3
Kentucky	22.6	36.2	8.9	22.7	36.3	9.1	20.4	35.8	6.1
Mississippi	25.7	41.3	11.4	29.8	45.7	14.0	20.2	35.5	7.5
Tennessee	20.9	32.3	10.1	21.7	33.3	10.7	17.1	27.8	7.7
West South Central	24.1	36.8	12.0	24.7	37.2	12.4	21.9	35.4	9.9
Arkansas	25.3	40.3	11.3	26.4	41.1	12.2	21.9	38.2	7.9
Louisiana	21.7	34.1	10.2	22.8	34.7	11.4	19.9	33.9	7.9
Oklahoma	28.0	41.1	15.2	27.4	40.4	14.7	34.4	50.4	19.9
Texas	23.8	36.1	11.9	24.3	36.5	12.2	21.1	33.1	10.4
Mountain	31.3	46.4	16.2	30.3	44.8	15.6	53.1	78.6	26.6
Arizona	30.1	44.7	15.3	28.1	41.5	14.6	49.0	76.2	21.1
Colorado	24.6	36.7	12.7	24.6	36.8	12.7	23.0	33.3	12.7*
Idaho	33.0	45.7	20.2	32.9	45.7	20.0	40.1*	38.9*	43.9*
Montana	38.0	57.7	17.7	35.9	55.2	16.2	103.4	136.3	68.5
Nevada	44.2	60.2	26.7	43.0	58.6	26.1	59.5	81.0	33.0*
New Mexico	37.4	58.0	16.5	35.2	54.2	15.8	66.9	108.3	25.0
Utah	25.1	34.3	16.3	24.3	33.2	16.0	61.9	86.0	37.6*
Wyoming	41.8	64.7	18.2	41.4	65.0	17.1	53.7*	49.1*	61.8*
Pacific	21.8	31.6	11.7	22.1	32.1	12.0	19.0	27.7	9.5
Alaska	14.5	17.9	9.5	16.1	19.8	10.3	8.8	9.8*	7.6*
California	22.2	32.3	11.9	22.3	32.5	12.1	20.2	30.5	9.4
Hawaii	12.1	17.7	5.1	14.1	20.8	4.8*	10.9	16.0	5.2
Oregon	26.3	38.2	14.7	25.9	38.0	14.3	44.9	49.9	39.0*
Washington	19.8	29.0	10.5	19.4	28.5	10.2	32.5	43.4	19.7

Table 27 Death rates for falls by age, color, and sex:
United States, 1959-61
(E900-E904)

Age	Total			White			Nonwhite		
	Total	Male	Female	Total	Male	Female	Total	Male	Female
All ages	10.5	10.5	10.5	11.0	10.8	11.2	6.7	8.8	4.7
Under 1	5.1	6.2	3.9	4.2	5.1	3.3	10.2	12.9	7.6
1	3.1	3.4	2.8	2.6	3.0	2.2	5.9	5.5	6.2
2	1.9	2.3	1.6	1.5	1.7	1.2	4.6	5.8	3.4
3	1.2	1.6	0.9	1.0	1.3	0.6	2.8	3.2	2.4
4	0.9	1.0	0.7	0.7	0.8	0.6	1.8	2.2*	1.4*
5 - 14	0.6	0.8	0.3	0.6	0.8	0.3	0.7	1.0	0.4
15 - 24	1.1	2.0	0.3	1.1	2.0	0.2	1.4	2.3	0.5
25 - 34	1.7	2.8	0.6	1.4	2.3	0.5	3.8	6.2	1.6
35 - 44	3.1	5.0	1.2	2.6	4.2	1.0	7.0	11.7	2.8
45 - 54	5.9	9.3	2.6	5.4	8.6	2.4	10.3	16.2	4.6
55 - 64	11.1	16.3	6.2	10.7	15.8	5.9	14.8	21.2	8.5
65 - 74	29.5	34.3	25.3	30.2	35.2	25.8	21.7	24.2	19.4
75 - 84	125.4	110.9	136.7	131.0	116.0	142.5	49.8	46.9	52.3
85 & over	510.8	428.0	563.6	541.2	457.7	593.7	146.1	114.8	170.5
Age-adjusted									
Total	7.8	9.1	6.5	7.8	8.9	6.6	7.1	9.6	4.7
Under 15	1.2	1.4	0.8	1.0	1.3	0.7	2.1	2.6	1.6
65 & over	73.2	69.6	75.2	76.3	72.7	78.2	33.8	33.6	33.8

Table 28   Percent distribution of deaths from falls, by place of occurrence and age: United States, 1959-61 (E900-E904)

Age	Total[a]	Home (.0)	Farm (.1)	Mine and quarry (.2)	Industrial place and premises (.3)	Place for recreation and sport (.4)	Street and highway (.5)	Public building (.6)	Resident institution (.7)	Other specified places (.8)
All ages	100.0	64.6	1.3	0.2	3.0	0.5	6.3	4.3	16.0	3.9
Under 1	100.0	96.7	0.4	-	-	0.4	0.7	0.5	0.7	0.5
1-4	100.0	91.0	1.3	-	0.1	1.0	2.0	1.1	0.6	2.9
5-14	100.0	47.8	5.5	0.9	2.4	9.2	7.0	5.9	2.0	19.3
15-24	100.0	15.7	3.8	1.7	16.2	7.9	8.3	8.0	4.1	34.3
25-34	100.0	30.8	3.2	1.7	18.4	1.6	11.3	9.7	4.7	18.6
35-44	100.0	41.9	2.0	0.9	13.3	1.2	12.8	11.3	4.7	11.9
45-54	100.0	48.3	2.5	0.5	10.8	0.6	12.3	9.7	5.6	9.7
55-64	100.0	52.7	2.6	0.3	7.8	0.4	11.6	8.7	9.2	6.7
65-74	100.0	65.6	1.6	0.0	1.4	0.2	8.6	5.2	14.6	2.8
75-84	100.0	70.6	0.7	0.0	0.3	0.1	4.6	2.4	20.3	1.0
85 & over	100.0	72.4	0.2	-	0.1	0.1	2.2	1.2	23.1	0.7

[a]Excludes place not specified.

Note: The decimal number under each place of occurrence in the column headings is a code used for non-transport accidents to denote the place where the accident occurred.

Table 29   Age-adjusted death rates for falls, by color and sex:
United States, each geographic division and state, 1959-61
(E900-E904)

Geographic area	Total			White			Nonwhite		
	Total	Male	Female	Total	Male	Female	Total	Male	Female
United States	7.8	9.1	6.5	7.8	8.9	6.6	7.1	9.6	4.7
New England	9.8	11.1	8.5	9.8	10.9	8.6	11.1	17.0	5.5
Connecticut	8.1	10.0	6.3	8.1	9.9	6.4	5.4*	8.0*	2.8*
Maine	6.1	6.7	5.4	6.1	6.7	5.5	8.1*	16.5*	-
Massachusetts	12.2	13.5	10.7	12.1	13.2	10.7	15.1	23.2	7.3*
New Hampshire	5.6	6.5	4.5	5.6	6.5	4.5	-	-	-
Rhode Island	8.7	9.4	7.7	8.6	9.3	7.7	13.4*	20.1*	6.7*
Vermont	7.4	8.2	6.8	7.4	8.2	6.8	-	-	-
Middle Atlantic	9.2	11.1	7.3	8.8	10.3	7.2	12.1	18.3	6.6
New Jersey	8.7	10.1	7.2	8.3	9.4	7.0	12.8	18.2	7.7
New York	9.6	11.9	7.4	9.1	10.9	7.3	13.1	20.4	6.9
Pennsylvania	8.7	10.3	7.2	8.6	9.9	7.2	9.9	14.7	5.5
East North Central	8.0	9.2	6.7	7.9	9.0	6.7	7.6	10.3	5.0
Illinois	6.5	8.3	4.7	6.3	7.9	4.7	7.0	11.1	3.2
Indiana	8.6	9.4	7.7	8.5	9.4	7.6	7.5	9.3	5.9
Michigan	8.5	9.5	7.3	8.4	9.3	7.4	8.0	10.5	5.5
Ohio	9.0	10.0	8.0	9.0	9.9	8.0	7.9	9.8	6.2
Wisconsin	7.6	8.6	6.6	7.6	8.6	6.5	7.7*	7.5*	8.3*
West North Central	7.6	8.7	6.4	7.4	8.5	6.2	11.4	13.6	9.3
Iowa	7.0	7.9	6.0	7.0	8.0	5.9	4.2*	1.3*	6.7*
Kansas	6.8	7.3	6.1	6.8	7.5	6.2	4.0*	4.5*	3.6*
Minnesota	7.5	8.8	6.2	7.5	8.8	6.2	9.9*	11.4*	8.2*
Missouri	8.4	9.5	7.3	7.9	8.8	6.9	13.9	16.9	11.1
Nebraska	7.7	9.6	5.7	7.6	9.5	5.7	11.8*	15.8*	7.2*
North Dakota	7.6	8.8	6.2	7.5	8.8	6.1	10.0*	8.1*	11.8*
South Dakota	6.5	8.2	4.8	6.4	8.0	4.7	8.1*	8.7*	7.6*
South Atlantic	6.8	7.7	5.8	6.7	7.5	5.9	6.4	8.4	4.6
Delaware	6.3	7.1	5.4	6.3	6.7	5.8	5.8*	9.6*	1.8*
District of Columbia	14.0	20.7	8.3	13.1	19.3	8.2	13.7	21.0	7.0
Florida	5.3	5.9	4.7	5.1	5.5	4.7	5.8	7.7	4.0
Georgia	6.3	6.7	5.7	6.4	6.8	5.9	5.9	6.7	5.1
Maryland	8.6	10.1	6.9	8.2	9.5	6.8	10.2	13.5	6.9
North Carolina	5.4	5.8	5.0	5.7	5.9	5.4	4.2	5.2	3.4
South Carolina	6.3	7.3	5.3	7.2	8.2	6.2	4.5	6.0	3.2
Virginia	7.9	8.8	6.9	8.3	9.0	7.4	6.0	7.7	4.3
West Virginia	7.6	9.1	6.2	7.7	9.2	6.2	6.6	7.3*	6.5*
East South Central	6.3	6.8	5.7	6.8	7.2	6.2	4.5	5.4	3.7
Alabama	5.5	6.0	4.9	5.9	6.3	5.3	4.5	5.5	3.8
Kentucky	8.6	9.1	8.0	8.8	9.4	8.0	7.0	6.3	7.5
Mississippi	4.7	5.2	4.2	5.3	5.5	5.0	3.7	4.7	2.9
Tennessee	5.8	6.4	5.2	6.1	6.5	5.5	4.4	6.0	3.0
West South Central	6.0	6.8	5.2	6.3	7.1	5.5	4.2	5.3	3.2
Arkansas	4.9	5.4	4.4	5.6	6.2	4.8	2.3	2.2*	2.5*
Louisiana	7.3	8.9	5.7	8.2	9.5	6.7	5.5	8.0	3.2
Oklahoma	7.1	8.2	6.0	7.2	8.2	6.1	6.0	7.6	4.6
Texas	5.5	6.0	4.8	5.7	6.3	5.0	3.5	3.9	3.1
Mountain	8.2	9.5	6.8	8.1	9.2	6.8	9.8	14.4	4.9
Arizona	5.9	7.8	4.0	5.6	7.2	3.9	8.6	12.3	4.8*
Colorado	9.1	10.9	7.4	9.1	10.7	7.5	9.3*	14.7*	4.0*
Idaho	8.0	9.0	6.8	7.9	9.0	6.8	9.1*	12.5*	4.0*
Montana	7.9	8.5	7.2	7.8	8.3	7.1	11.8*	14.7*	8.0*
Nevada	9.2	9.5	8.7	9.2	9.3	8.8	9.3*	13.1*	4.0*
New Mexico	7.7	8.9	6.4	7.7	8.7	6.5	8.4*	13.1*	3.7*
Utah	8.8	9.6	7.7	8.6	9.2	7.8	17.2*	29.0*	-
Wyoming	10.3	10.8	9.8	10.2	10.8	9.4	25.2*	14.1*	42.5*
Pacific	7.1	8.7	5.5	7.1	8.7	5.6	6.0	8.2	3.4
Alaska	7.9	8.2	7.5*	7.8	8.8*	6.3*	8.4*	6.3*	10.7*
California	7.3	8.7	5.7	7.2	8.7	5.7	6.6	9.0	3.9
Hawaii	4.1	5.7	2.2*	4.7	5.2*	4.0*	3.8	5.9	1.3*
Oregon	5.8	7.4	4.2	5.8	7.4	4.2	7.6*	9.8*	5.5*
Washington	7.7	9.7	5.7	7.7	9.6	5.7	7.9	10.7*	3.9*

Table 30   Age-adjusted death rates for falls, persons age 65 and over,
by color and sex: United States, each geographic division and state, 1959-61
(E900-E904)

Geographic area	Total			White			Nonwhite		
	Total	Male	Female	Total	Male	Female	Total	Male	Female
United States	73.2	69.6	75.2	76.3	72.7	78.2	33.8	33.6	33.8
New England	97.3	90.5	100.6	97.6	90.6	101.1	71.8	89.3*	56.4*
Connecticut	75.9	78.7	72.4	76.8	79.6	73.1	30.2*	33.1*	27.9*
Maine	54.2	49.0	57.8	54.1	48.6	57.9	118.6*	240.6*	-
Massachusetts	122.6	111.9	128.3	123.1	111.9	129.0	93.8	113.0*	76.4*
New Hampshire	55.2	48.8	58.6	55.4	49.0	58.6	-	-	-
Rhode Island	85.8	77.4	90.4	86.0	77.0	91.0	73.6*	104.0*	41.7*
Vermont	80.5	88.1	74.8	80.7	88.3	74.9	-	-	-
Middle Atlantic	82.9	81.5	82.9	84.3	82.5	84.6	47.7	56.1	40.0
New Jersey	79.7	75.6	81.7	81.2	76.7	83.6	49.1	55.7	41.9*
New York	82.3	81.8	81.6	83.7	82.9	83.3	45.0	53.3	38.1
Pennsylvania	85.2	83.8	85.3	86.7	84.8	87.1	50.6	60.4	41.7
East North Central	78.0	75.3	79.1	79.6	76.9	80.7	38.1	40.8	35.5
Illinois	53.3	56.7	50.2	55.0	58.2	52.1	22.9	32.7	14.8*
Indiana	90.0	84.0	93.9	91.7	85.7	95.6	39.6	39.6*	40.4*
Michigan	85.5	80.4	88.1	87.1	81.4	90.0	48.9	56.2	42.5
Ohio	92.4	86.0	96.0	94.6	88.4	97.9	47.5	42.6	51.9
Wisconsin	77.8	76.1	78.0	78.0	76.7	78.0	40.5*	-	88.4*
West North Central	73.7	71.5	74.8	74.2	72.1	75.2	57.4	49.8	63.8
Iowa	72.2	71.0	72.2	72.7	71.6	72.5	8.4*	-	15.1*
Kansas	67.3	62.1	71.1	68.3	63.0	72.1	39.8*	40.3*	39.6*
Minnesota	73.3	74.3	71.7	73.5	74.7	71.7	43.3*	20.4*	65.8*
Missouri	79.2	73.8	82.8	79.8	74.8	83.1	67.9	59.2	75.0
Nebraska	76.9	82.0	71.7	77.2	82.3	72.2	52.4*	58.6*	39.8*
North Dakota	75.5	68.3	82.9	76.2	68.9	83.7	-	-	-
South Dakota	54.4	52.7	55.9	54.4	53.3	55.4	64.8*	40.5*	92.5*
South Atlantic	60.4	54.8	64.5	66.3	60.3	70.6	30.4	28.5	31.9
Delaware	61.4	51.6	69.1	65.3	54.0	74.0	26.2*	33.7*	17.9*
District of Columbia	79.3	86.3	72.9	92.2	105.3	81.8	47.7	46.5*	48.3*
Florida	46.7	42.5	50.4	49.2	44.4	53.3	24.5	26.4*	22.6*
Georgia	56.4	48.7	61.6	68.2	60.6	73.1	22.7	16.7*	27.2
Maryland	77.4	73.7	79.2	79.9	75.8	82.1	58.2	61.5	55.4
North Carolina	52.8	45.7	57.9	59.3	51.1	65.2	26.0	24.4	26.7
South Carolina	58.7	51.8	63.4	75.1	68.9	79.3	22.0	19.0*	24.4
Virginia	77.6	71.5	81.5	86.5	80.8	89.7	36.1	33.8	38.1
West Virginia	65.8	62.1	68.5	66.7	63.9	68.6	43.2*	25.7*	63.0*
East South Central	61.0	51.2	68.5	70.3	60.2	77.8	25.4	18.5	31.3
Alabama	51.1	42.2	57.7	61.5	53.2	67.4	25.4	15.8*	32.8
Kentucky	86.1	75.1	94.3	90.4	79.5	98.6	33.1	24.1*	40.7*
Mississippi	43.4	35.2	50.0	56.5	47.1	63.3	23.3	17.8	28.4
Tennessee	55.7	45.4	64.0	61.3	50.3	69.9	24.9	20.9*	28.7
West South Central	58.5	53.4	62.1	64.7	59.8	68.0	24.5	21.2	27.3
Arkansas	51.4	45.7	56.4	59.6	55.9	62.5	19.1	7.5*	30.5
Louisiana	62.4	57.9	65.3	78.6	72.2	82.5	28.5	30.8	26.1
Oklahoma	69.8	64.2	73.9	72.4	67.1	76.4	39.0	34.7*	43.2*
Texas	55.0	50.2	58.4	59.6	55.1	62.6	20.0	16.5	23.2
Mountain	74.7	69.6	78.4	75.4	69.9	79.4	56.1	63.4	46.0*
Arizona	42.1	40.0	43.8	42.2	40.4	43.5	41.2*	34.4*	50.9*
Colorado	80.6	81.7	78.8	81.3	81.8	80.0	43.9*	77.0*	12.6*
Idaho	82.3	82.1	82.1	82.0	81.4	82.3	107.1*	128.6*	58.6*
Montana	75.8	68.0	82.8	76.6	67.9	84.7	45.3*	82.6*	-
Nevada	97.8	89.5	104.6	99.4	90.4	107.0	71.7*	88.6*	40.8*
New Mexico	75.6	62.8	87.4	77.8	65.1	89.4	40.1*	31.8*	49.2*
Utah	83.2	68.5	94.5	82.5	65.5	95.4	129.3*	191.1	-
Wyoming	84.9	70.8	98.9	82.6	72.0	92.7	254.2*	-	620.8*
Pacific	63.4	63.1	62.8	64.5	64.1	64.1	37.4	46.9	25.9
Alaska	78.2*	70.2*	91.4*	78.3*	81.4*	78.0*	75.7*	37.6*	118.7*
California	65.4	64.9	64.7	66.3	65.5	65.8	41.9	52.4	30.2
Hawaii	21.0	29.3*	11.1*	17.9*	21.7*	15.3*	22.0*	31.0*	9.3*
Oregon	49.2	50.8	47.9	49.5	51.1	48.3	18.0*	31.9*	-
Washington	66.6	66.0	66.4	66.9	66.2	66.9	46.7*	57.9*	26.3*

Table 31   Death rates for fire and explosion, by age, color, and sex:
                                        United States, 1959-61
                                              (E916)

Age	Total			White			Nonwhite		
	Total	Male	Female	Total	Male	Female	Total	Male	Female
All ages	4.0	4.6	3.4	3.2	3.8	2.5	10.7	10.9	10.4
Under 1	6.8	7.0	6.6	3.5	3.3	3.7	25.7	28.4	23.0
1	6.1	6.3	6.0	3.8	4.0	3.6	19.8	19.8	19.8
2	6.9	7.1	6.8	4.3	4.5	4.0	22.6	22.4	22.7
3	6.6	6.4	6.9	4.0	4.3	3.7	22.3	19.2	25.3
4	6.2	5.2	7.2	3.7	3.4	4.1	21.0	16.1	25.8
5 - 14	2.2	1.8	2.6	1.5	1.4	1.6	6.5	4.4	8.7
15 - 24	1.3	1.7	0.9	1.1	1.4	0.7	2.7	3.2	2.3
25 - 34	2.3	3.2	1.4	1.9	2.7	1.1	4.9	6.5	3.6
35 - 44	2.9	4.0	1.9	2.4	3.4	1.5	7.0	9.3	5.0
45 - 54	4.2	5.5	2.9	3.7	4.8	2.5	9.1	12.2	6.2
55 - 64	4.9	6.1	3.7	4.0	5.2	2.8	14.0	15.1	13.1
65 - 74	8.1	9.6	6.8	6.5	8.1	5.1	26.3	26.4	26.1
75 - 84	17.0	20.7	14.1	14.6	18.5	11.6	50.2	48.3	51.9
85 & over	30.7	39.9	24.8	25.9	35.6	19.9	87.9	86.1	89.4
Age-adjusted									
Total	3.6	4.3	2.9	2.8	3.5	2.1	9.7	10.4	9.2
Under 15	3.6	3.3	3.9	2.3	2.2	2.4	11.5	9.7	13.3
65 & over	11.3	13.6	9.4	9.3	11.8	7.3	34.8	34.3	35.2

Table 32   Age-adjusted death rates for fire and explosion,
by color and sex: United States,
each geographic division and state, 1959-61
(E916)

Geographic area	Total			White			Nonwhite		
	Total	Male	Female	Total	Male	Female	Total	Male	Female
United States	3.6	4.3	2.9	2.8	3.5	2.1	9.7	10.4	9.2
New England	3.0	3.7	2.3	2.8	3.6	2.2	9.1	9.9	8.5
Connecticut	2.5	3.1	1.9	2.2	2.9	1.7	7.5	8.1*	6.8*
Maine	5.3	7.1	3.7	5.3	6.9	3.7	26.5*	50.6*	-
Massachusetts	2.8	3.4	2.3	2.6	3.2	2.1	9.3	10.0	8.6
New Hampshire	3.2	4.0	2.6	3.2	4.0	2.5	8.9*	-	20.3*
Rhode Island	2.7	3.5	2.1	2.5	3.4	1.7	12.3*	9.1*	16.7*
Vermont	3.4	4.3	2.5*	3.3	4.2	2.5*	23.1*	48.1*	-
Middle Atlantic	2.7	3.3	2.3	2.3	2.8	1.9	7.2	8.2	6.4
New Jersey	2.8	3.4	2.1	2.2	2.7	1.7	8.6	10.8	6.5
New York	2.8	3.2	2.3	2.4	2.8	2.0	6.4	7.2	5.7
Pennsylvania	2.7	3.2	2.3	2.3	2.8	1.9	7.8	8.2	7.5
East North Central	2.8	3.5	2.1	2.5	3.1	1.9	6.6	8.2	5.0
Illinois	2.9	3.5	2.3	2.5	3.1	1.9	6.2	7.2	5.2
Indiana	3.2	4.5	1.9	3.0	4.2	1.8	6.7	9.3	4.3
Michigan	2.8	3.6	2.0	2.5	3.2	1.7	6.1	7.6	4.5
Ohio	2.7	3.4	2.1	2.3	2.9	1.8	7.4	9.3	5.6
Wisconsin	2.2	2.7	1.9	2.1	2.5	1.8	6.5	10.4*	2.4*
West North Central	2.8	3.6	2.1	2.6	3.3	1.8	10.1	10.6	9.8
Iowa	2.1	2.4	1.8	2.1	2.4	1.8	8.4*	4.5*	12.4*
Kansas	3.0	4.0	2.0	2.8	3.8	1.8	7.1	6.8*	7.4*
Minnesota	2.3	2.8	1.8	2.1	2.7	1.7	11.7*	11.7*	11.9*
Missouri	3.6	4.6	2.7	3.0	3.9	2.0	10.2	10.8	9.7
Nebraska	2.6	3.6	1.7	2.4	3.4	1.5	9.4*	10.8*	8.1*
North Dakota	3.7	5.2	2.1	3.5	5.0	1.9	10.6*	13.0*	8.5*
South Dakota	3.1	4.1	2.1	2.4	3.2	1.6*	21.3*	30.4*	12.7*
South Atlantic	4.9	5.7	4.2	3.1	3.9	2.4	11.4	12.4	10.5
Delaware	4.8	6.3	3.3	3.0	3.8	2.1*	16.4	22.6*	10.3*
District of Columbia	4.9	5.2	4.7	3.9	3.9	4.0	5.8	6.3	5.4
Florida	3.6	4.0	3.2	2.2	2.6	1.7	11.3	11.9	10.7
Georgia	5.9	6.4	5.6	3.6	4.2	3.1	11.9	12.4	11.7
Maryland	4.1	5.2	3.2	2.6	3.3	1.9	12.1	14.6	9.5
North Carolina	5.1	6.4	4.0	3.4	4.7	2.1	10.5	11.8	9.4
South Carolina	7.3	8.1	6.6	3.5	5.1	2.1	14.5	14.4	14.7
Virginia	4.5	5.3	3.6	2.8	3.6	2.2	11.0	13.1	8.9
West Virginia	5.3	6.4	4.2	5.0	6.3	3.8	9.9	8.6*	11.8
East South Central	5.9	6.6	5.4	3.9	4.8	3.0	12.9	12.8	13.2
Alabama	6.5	7.1	5.9	3.8	4.6	2.9	12.7	13.3	12.3
Kentucky	4.7	5.7	3.7	3.9	4.9	2.9	14.4	15.3	13.5
Mississippi	8.3	7.8	8.9	4.0	4.5	3.5	13.8	12.4	15.3
Tennessee	5.1	6.0	4.2	3.9	4.9	3.0	10.9	11.4	10.5
West South Central	5.3	6.1	4.5	3.9	4.9	3.0	11.8	12.1	11.7
Arkansas	6.8	7.9	5.8	4.0	4.5	3.4	16.5	20.3	13.2
Louisiana	5.8	5.7	5.9	3.5	4.1	2.8	10.7	9.0	12.3
Oklahoma	5.2	6.5	3.9	4.2	5.5	3.0	14.8	17.7	12.4
Texas	4.9	5.7	4.0	4.0	5.0	3.0	10.7	10.9	10.7
Mountain	3.1	4.1	2.0	2.8	3.9	1.7	7.9	6.3	9.7
Arizona	4.1	5.1	3.1	3.3	4.7	2.0	10.8	8.0	14.0
Colorado	2.0	2.8	1.4	2.0	2.8	1.2	3.9*	3.4*	4.5*
Idaho	2.5	3.7	1.2*	2.5	3.8	1.2*	-	-	-
Montana	2.9	4.1	1.7	2.8	4.0	1.5*	6.9*	5.2*	8.9*
Nevada	4.3	5.0	3.6*	4.0	4.6*	3.5*	7.7*	9.8*	5.5*
New Mexico	4.4	6.1	2.6	4.2	6.0	2.4	5.3*	5.8*	4.8*
Utah	2.0	2.5	1.6	1.9	2.4	1.3	13.4*	4.1*	28.6*
Wyoming	4.0	5.6	2.2*	3.8	5.5	2.0*	13.8*	11.9*	17.6*
Pacific	2.9	3.7	2.2	2.7	3.5	2.0	4.5	5.3	3.5
Alaska	12.8	14.4	10.3	7.3	10.0	2.7*	30.3	28.0	33.1
California	2.7	3.4	2.1	2.6	3.3	2.0	4.1	5.2	2.9
Hawaii	1.8	2.3	1.2*	2.7*	3.8*	1.5*	1.4*	1.7*	1.0*
Oregon	3.4	4.5	2.3	3.3	4.4	2.3	6.8*	8.5*	5.3*
Washington	3.0	4.1	1.9	2.8	3.8	1.8	8.0	9.7*	5.2*

Table 33   Death rates for drowning, by age, color, and sex:
United States, 1959-61
(E929)

Age	Total			White			Nonwhite		
	Total	Male	Female	Total	Male	Female	Total	Male	Female
All ages	2.9	4.9	0.9	2.6	4.3	0.9	5.3	9.8	1.1
Under 1	1.4	1.4	1.4	1.4	1.3	1.4	1.5	1.7*	1.3*
1	6.1	7.1	5.0	6.5	7.7	5.3	3.4	3.8	2.9
2	4.5	6.0	2.9	4.9	6.5	3.1	2.1	2.7	1.6*
3	3.5	5.1	1.8	3.7	5.5	1.9	1.8	2.8	0.9*
4	2.7	4.1	1.3	2.9	4.4	1.4	1.3	2.1*	0.6*
5 - 14	3.6	5.9	1.2	3.1	4.9	1.2	7.0	12.5	1.4
15 - 24	4.7	8.7	0.7	4.0	7.4	0.7	9.4	18.4	1.0
25 - 34	2.1	3.9	0.4	1.7	3.2	0.3	4.8	9.6	0.7
35 - 44	1.9	3.4	0.5	1.6	2.9	0.4	4.5	8.2	1.1
45 - 54	2.0	3.5	0.5	1.8	3.1	0.5	3.8	7.3	0.6*
55 - 64	2.1	3.8	0.6	1.9	3.4	0.6	4.3	7.7	0.9*
65 - 74	2.1	3.7	0.6	2.0	3.6	0.6	3.0	5.1	1.1*
75 - 84	2.1	3.9	0.7	1.9	3.7	0.6	4.0	6.9	1.4*
85 & over	2.8	4.8	1.5	2.7	4.5	1.6	3.7*	7.4*	0.8*
Age-adjusted									
Total	2.9	5.1	0.8	2.6	4.4	0.8	5.5	10.2	1.0
Under 15	3.6	5.6	1.6	3.4	4.9	1.6	5.5	9.4	1.4
65 & over	2.1	3.8	0.7	2.0	3.7	0.6	3.3	5.6	1.2

Table 34

Death rates for drowning, by age: United States,
each geographic division and state, 1959-61
(E929)

Geographic area	All ages	Under 5	5-14	15-24	25-34	35-44	45-54	55-64	65-74	75-84	85 & over
United States	2.9	3.6	3.6	4.7	2.1	1.9	2.0	2.1	2.1	2.1	2.8
New England	2.5	3.3	3.6	3.5	1.7	1.6	1.5	1.7	2.3	2.3	2.4*
Connecticut	2.2	2.2*	2.5	4.0	1.9*	1.3*	1.2*	1.6*	2.9*	1.5*	4.7*
Maine	3.5	4.3*	4.9	4.7*	2.6*	2.5*	2.5*	3.4*	1.5*	3.1*	4.3*
Massachusetts	2.4	2.7	3.7	3.0	1.7	1.6	1.6	1.9	2.5	2.7*	0.9*
New Hampshire	3.1	7.1*	4.9*	4.2*	0.9*	1.7*	1.0*	0.6*	1.6*	5.0*	7.0*
Rhode Island	1.7	3.7*	3.7*	1.4*	0.3*	1.4*	1.0*	0.4*	1.1*	-	-
Vermont	3.0	8.4*	3.4*	6.2*	0.8*	2.8*	-	-	1.2*	-	-
Middle Atlantic	2.2	2.3	2.7	3.6	1.5	1.5	1.7	2.0	2.3	1.9	2.9*
New Jersey	2.4	2.6	3.4	4.2	1.2	1.0	1.6	2.4	2.2	3.0*	2.4*
New York	2.4	2.3	2.5	3.6	1.8	1.9	2.2	2.2	2.7	2.2	4.8*
Pennsylvania	1.9	2.2	2.6	3.4	1.2	1.3	1.2	1.6	1.8	1.0*	0.5*
East North Central	2.3	2.6	3.4	3.8	1.6	1.2	1.4	1.6	1.8	2.0	3.2*
Illinois	2.3	1.9	3.0	4.2	1.6	1.6	1.8	2.0	1.9	2.2*	3.2*
Indiana	2.3	2.6	3.9	3.4	1.7	1.4	1.6	0.6*	1.2*	1.5*	2.4*
Michigan	2.5	3.2	3.1	4.2	2.1	1.3	1.4	1.5	2.1	2.9*	2.0*
Ohio	2.2	2.2	3.7	3.4	1.4	0.9	0.9	1.6	1.9	1.2*	3.2*
Wisconsin	2.3	4.0	3.3	3.4	0.9*	0.8*	1.6	1.4*	1.8*	2.3*	5.9*
West North Central	2.4	3.2	3.4	4.2	1.8	1.4	1.5	1.2	1.5	1.6	2.7*
Iowa	2.2	2.7	3.7	3.3	1.6*	1.4*	2.0*	0.9*	1.5*	0.7*	-
Kansas	2.4	2.4*	4.0	4.1	1.5*	1.3*	1.3*	1.2*	1.8*	2.7*	4.0*
Minnesota	2.5	3.8	3.2	4.9	1.8	1.4*	0.9*	1.7*	1.6*	1.0*	1.6*
Missouri	2.3	2.5	3.0	4.0	1.8	1.5	1.6	1.2*	1.4*	1.3*	4.1*
Nebraska	2.3	4.2	2.8	3.6	1.8*	1.8*	1.5*	0.5*	1.0*	2.7*	6.4*
North Dakota	3.4	4.2*	5.1	3.7*	2.3*	1.8*	2.4*	2.6*	2.6*	3.8*	-
South Dakota	3.0	4.8*	2.8*	6.2*	3.4*	0.8*	2.4*	0.6*	2.1*	1.6*	-
South Atlantic	3.9	4.1	4.4	6.3	3.0	2.9	3.1	3.2	2.6	2.2	2.1*
Delaware	3.6	4.8*	3.4*	5.8*	1.6*	3.1*	2.7*	6.8*	1.4*	-	-
District of Columbia	2.8	1.7*	2.3*	2.7*	2.1*	4.1*	3.7*	1.8*	1.4*	8.9*	-
Florida	5.7	11.0	6.1	7.4	3.8	3.4	5.3	5.0	4.3	3.6*	4.2*
Georgia	3.6	3.2	5.0	5.4	3.1	3.2	2.6	2.0*	1.7*	0.4*	2.1*
Maryland	2.6	2.0	3.0	4.5	2.1	1.8	1.6*	3.1	2.0*	3.2*	2.7*
North Carolina	3.4	2.5	3.2	6.8	2.5	3.3	2.4	2.6	1.4*	2.7*	-
South Carolina	4.9	1.6*	6.2	8.8	4.3	3.9	3.4	4.3	2.3*	0.8*	4.0*
Virginia	3.2	3.0	3.5	5.9	2.9	2.1	2.3	2.5	1.7*	0.4*	-
West Virginia	3.5	2.5*	4.6	6.6	2.2*	2.8	2.5*	1.5*	3.6*	0.7*	-
East South Central	3.2	2.5	4.3	5.9	2.6	2.4	2.0	2.3	1.3	2.2	3.8*
Alabama	3.2	2.0	3.9	6.2	2.9	2.0	1.6*	3.1	1.5*	2.7*	2.3*
Kentucky	3.0	2.9	3.3	5.8	2.4	2.2	1.6*	1.6*	1.2*	3.1*	3.8*
Mississippi	5.1	4.4	6.5	7.1	4.8	4.6	4.2	3.9	1.3*	1.9*	8.6*
Tennessee	2.4	1.1*	3.9	4.8	1.5	1.7	1.5*	1.4*	1.0*	1.1*	1.9*
West South Central	3.6	3.7	4.8	6.1	2.6	2.4	2.2	2.5	2.0	2.2	1.6*
Arkansas	3.7	2.4*	5.3	7.0	2.1*	2.9*	2.7*	2.0*	3.1*	1.2*	3.0*
Louisiana	4.1	3.0	5.0	8.3	3.7	2.4	2.4	2.8	1.4*	3.0	-
Oklahoma	2.9	4.0	3.4	4.3	2.5	1.7*	1.5*	2.6*	3.0*	3.1*	-
Texas	3.5	4.0	4.9	5.7	2.4	2.4	2.1	2.4	1.5	1.9*	2.3*
Mountain	3.9	9.7	3.7	4.6	2.8	2.1	2.0	2.3	2.8	2.2*	3.4*
Arizona	4.9	13.6	2.9	5.4	4.5	3.5*	1.5*	3.2*	4.7*	3.0*	8.1*
Colorado	2.6	4.9	3.7	3.8	1.6*	1.3*	1.1*	1.2*	1.3*	0.7*	-
Idaho	6.1	19.5	4.7	8.5	2.2*	2.0*	2.8*	4.7*	2.7*	1.9*	-
Montana	5.8	12.8	5.6	6.3*	5.8*	3.5*	4.1*	3.2*	4.7*	3.5*	-
Nevada	3.9	10.1*	1.8*	5.3*	4.1*	1.5*	3.7*	1.5*	2.6*	7.0*	-
New Mexico	3.6	6.9	5.0	2.5*	2.8*	2.0*	1.1*	3.0*	1.9*	2.5*	-
Utah	3.0	7.1	2.4*	3.9*	0.9*	1.6*	2.4*	0.6*	3.4*	1.9*	10.3*
Wyoming	3.0	9.9*	1.9*	3.0*	1.5*	1.5*	2.8*	1.3*	-	4.8*	25.3*
Pacific	3.1	5.6	2.8	4.1	2.3	2.2	2.6	2.7	2.2	2.7	3.2*
Alaska	11.9	6.8*	13.0*	13.1*	7.6*	13.5*	12.3*	29.2*	-	24.6*	-
California	2.6	5.5	2.4	3.2	1.8	1.9	2.1	2.0	1.8	2.2	3.1*
Hawaii	5.0	5.4*	2.2*	7.6	4.3*	4.1*	5.0*	9.7*	3.4*	12.6*	21.1*
Oregon	4.6	7.7	3.9	9.0	2.5*	2.5*	4.2	4.4	2.5*	3.1*	3.3*
Washington	3.9	5.4	3.9	4.4	4.1	2.7	3.6	3.1	3.9	3.2*	2.1*

Table 35   Age-adjusted death rates for drowning, by color and sex:
United States, each geographic division and state, 1959-61
(E929)

Geographic area	Total			White			Nonwhite		
	Total	Male	Female	Total	Male	Female	Total	Male	Female
United States	2.9	5.1	0.8	2.6	4.4	0.8	5.5	10.2	1.0
New England	2.5	4.2	0.9	2.4	4.0	0.8	6.1	10.3	2.0*
Connecticut	2.3	3.8	0.8	1.9	3.2	0.7	8.9	14.8	3.3*
Maine	3.5	5.9	1.2	3.5	5.8	1.1*	13.2*	17.1*	10.0*
Massachusetts	2.4	4.2	0.7	2.4	4.1	0.7	3.9*	7.5*	0.4*
New Hampshire	2.9	4.3	1.5*	2.9	4.3	1.5*	-	-	-
Rhode Island	1.6	2.6	0.6*	1.6	2.5	0.6*	2.6*	3.1*	1.6*
Vermont	3.0	4.6	1.4*	3.0	4.6	1.4*	-	-	-
Middle Atlantic	2.3	4.1	0.6	2.1	3.6	0.6	4.6	8.7	0.9
New Jersey	2.4	4.3	0.6	2.1	3.8	0.6	5.2	10.1	0.8*
New York	2.4	4.3	0.7	2.2	3.8	0.6	4.9	9.4	1.1
Pennsylvania	2.0	3.5	0.6	1.9	3.3	0.6	3.5	6.5	0.7*
East North Central	2.3	4.1	0.6	2.2	3.9	0.6	3.4	6.2	0.7
Illinois	2.4	4.3	0.7	2.3	4.1	0.6	3.5	6.1	1.0*
Indiana	2.3	4.0	0.6	2.1	3.7	0.6	4.6	8.5	0.9*
Michigan	2.5	4.4	0.7	2.5	4.4	0.7	2.6	4.7	0.6*
Ohio	2.1	3.9	0.4	2.0	3.6	0.5	3.6	7.0	0.3*
Wisconsin	2.2	3.7	0.8	2.2	3.6	0.8	3.4*	6.2*	0.5*
West North Central	2.5	4.2	0.7	2.4	4.0	0.7	4.4	8.5	0.7*
Iowa	2.3	4.2	0.4*	2.2	4.0	0.4*	10.4*	21.6*	-
Kansas	2.4	4.2	0.6	2.4	4.1	0.7	3.3*	6.7*	-
Minnesota	2.6	4.2	1.0	2.5	4.0	1.0	10.0*	18.6*	1.1*
Missouri	2.3	4.0	0.7	2.3	4.0	0.7	2.6	5.0	0.5*
Nebraska	2.3	3.8	0.9	2.3	3.7	0.8*	4.4*	5.4*	3.4*
North Dakota	3.2	5.0	1.3*	2.9	4.6	1.2*	19.6*	28.9*	9.4*
South Dakota	3.1	5.5	0.7*	2.6	4.4	0.7*	15.7*	32.1*	-
South Atlantic	3.9	6.9	1.0	3.1	5.2	1.0	6.7	12.7	1.0
Delaware	3.6	6.5	0.8*	3.1	5.5	0.8*	7.0*	12.8*	1.2*
District of Columbia	2.7	5.3	0.5*	2.6	4.5	0.9*	2.8	5.8	0.1*
Florida	5.7	9.6	1.9	4.6	7.3	1.8	10.9	19.9	2.3
Georgia	3.6	6.1	1.2	2.9	4.6	1.3	5.3	10.2	0.9
Maryland	2.7	4.8	0.6	2.2	3.7	0.7	5.2	10.0	0.4*
North Carolina	3.5	6.1	0.8	2.7	4.6	0.8	5.7	11.0	0.8*
South Carolina	4.9	9.1	0.7	2.9	5.1	0.6*	8.9	17.5	1.0*
Virginia	3.2	5.7	0.7	2.6	4.4	0.7	5.9	11.0	0.8*
West Virginia	3.5	6.4	0.7	3.4	6.2	0.8	5.7*	11.3*	0.5*
East South Central	3.3	5.8	0.8	2.7	4.6	0.7	5.4	10.2	1.1
Alabama	3.3	6.0	0.7	2.3	4.3	0.4*	5.5	10.2	1.2
Kentucky	3.0	5.3	0.7	2.8	4.9	0.8	5.6	11.0	0.3*
Mississippi	5.1	8.9	1.5	4.1	6.6	1.6	6.4	12.2	1.2
Tennessee	2.5	4.4	0.6	2.2	3.8	0.5	3.9	7.2	0.9*
West South Central	3.6	6.2	0.9	3.1	5.3	0.9	5.8	10.8	1.0
Arkansas	3.8	6.5	1.1	3.4	5.7	1.1	5.1	9.4	1.2*
Louisiana	4.2	7.7	0.8	3.1	5.6	0.8	6.3	12.2	0.9*
Oklahoma	2.9	5.1	0.8	2.7	4.8	0.7	4.7	8.8	1.0*
Texas	3.5	6.0	1.0	3.2	5.4	1.0	5.6	10.5	1.1
Mountain	3.6	5.9	1.3	3.3	5.4	1.3	9.9	16.9	2.5*
Arizona	4.5	7.3	1.8	4.0	6.6	1.5	9.7	15.4	3.2*
Colorado	2.5	4.2	0.7	2.4	4.0	0.8	4.7*	9.3*	-
Idaho	5.4	8.4	2.4	5.2	7.9	2.4	21.3*	41.2*	-
Montana	5.6	9.0	2.1	5.0	8.0	2.1	19.6*	36.5*	1.3*
Nevada	3.8	5.2	2.3*	2.8	4.1*	1.5*	17.1*	18.9*	15.2*
New Mexico	3.1	5.5	0.7*	2.7	4.7	0.8*	7.9*	15.5*	-
Utah	2.6	4.2	1.0*	2.5	4.1	1.0*	6.0*	10.0*	2.0*
Wyoming	2.7	4.5	0.8*	2.6	4.3	0.8*	13.9*	24.4*	-
Pacific	3.0	5.1	1.0	2.8	4.6	1.0	5.5	9.4	1.3
Alaska	12.5	19.3	2.5*	7.5	11.4	1.6*	30.6	51.5	4.6*
California	2.5	4.1	1.0	2.4	3.9	1.0	3.9	6.7	1.0
Hawaii	5.3	8.5	1.3*	6.5	9.7	1.9*	4.7	7.8	1.0*
Oregon	4.7	7.9	1.6	4.5	7.6	1.4	15.4*	20.1*	10.8*
Washington	3.9	6.7	0.9	3.5	6.1	0.9	12.7	22.6	1.2*

Table 36   Death rates for firearm accidents, by age, color, and sex:
United States, 1959-61
(E919)

Age	Total			White			Nonwhite		
	Total	Male	Female	Total	Male	Female	Total	Male	Female
All ages	1.3	2.2	0.3	1.2	2.1	0.3	2.0	3.3	0.8
Under 1	0.2	0.2*	0.2*	0.1*	0.1*	0.1*	0.5*	0.5*	0.4*
1 - 4	0.5	0.6	0.4	0.4	0.5	0.3	1.0	1.2	0.9
5 - 14	1.2	2.1	0.4	1.2	2.0	0.3	1.8	2.8	0.8
15 - 24	2.4	4.4	0.5	2.2	4.0	0.4	4.0	6.8	1.4
25 - 34	1.4	2.3	0.4	1.2	2.1	0.4	2.4	4.1	0.9
35 - 44	1.1	2.0	0.3	1.1	1.9	0.3	1.7	3.0	0.5
45 - 54	1.4	2.5	0.2	1.3	2.5	0.2	1.9	3.3	0.6
55 - 64	1.1	2.2	0.1	1.1	2.1	0.1	1.3	2.4	0.2*
65 - 74	0.7	1.4	0.1*	0.7	1.4	0.1*	1.0	1.9	0.1*
75 - 84	0.7	1.5	0.2*	0.7	1.4	0.2*	0.9*	1.8*	0.2*
85 & over	0.4*	0.7*	0.1*	0.4*	0.8*	0.1*	-	-	-

Table 37   Death rates for accidental poisoning, by type of poisoning,
                  age, color and sex: United States, 1959-61

Type of poisoning and age	Total			White			Nonwhite		
	Total	Male	Female	Total	Male	Female	Total	Male	Female
Solid and liquid substances (E870-E888)									
All ages	1.0	1.2	0.7	0.8	1.0	0.6	2.1	2.8	1.5
Under 1	1.3	1.5	1.1	1.0	1.0	0.9	3.2	4.0	2.4
1 - 4	2.4	2.7	2.2	1.7	1.8	1.6	6.8	7.7	5.8
5 - 14	0.1	0.1	0.1	0.1	0.1	0.1	0.2	0.2*	0.2*
15 - 24	0.4	0.5	0.2	0.3	0.5	0.2	0.7	1.1	0.4*
25 - 34	0.8	0.9	0.6	0.6	0.7	0.5	2.1	2.6	1.6
35 - 44	1.3	1.6	1.0	1.1	1.2	0.9	3.3	4.6	2.0
45 - 54	1.6	2.0	1.1	1.5	1.9	1.1	2.5	3.7	1.3
55 - 64	1.2	1.6	0.8	1.1	1.5	0.8	1.8	2.7	1.0
65 - 74	1.0	1.2	0.7	1.0	1.2	0.8	1.2	1.9	0.4*
75 - 84	0.8	1.0	0.7	0.8	1.0	0.7	1.0*	1.1*	1.0*
85 & over	1.2	1.3*	1.1*	1.2	1.2*	1.1*	1.4*	2.1*	0.8*
Gases and vapors (E890-E895)									
All ages	0.7	1.0	0.4	0.6	1.0	0.3	0.8	1.1	0.6
Under 1	0.4	0.4	0.4	0.4	0.3*	0.4	0.7*	0.9*	0.4*
1 - 4	0.2	0.2	0.2	0.2	0.2	0.2	0.3	0.3*	0.3*
5 - 14	0.1	0.2	0.1	0.1	0.2	0.1	0.2	0.2*	0.2*
15 - 24	0.8	1.1	0.5	0.8	1.1	0.5	0.8	0.9	0.7
25 - 34	0.7	1.1	0.3	0.7	1.1	0.3	1.2	1.7	0.8
35 - 44	0.7	1.2	0.3	0.7	1.1	0.2	1.1	1.6	0.8
45 - 54	1.0	1.6	0.4	0.9	1.5	0.3	1.3	2.0	0.7
55 - 64	1.1	1.7	0.4	1.0	1.7	0.4	1.5	2.0	0.9
65 - 74	1.1	1.6	0.6	1.1	1.6	0.6	1.4	2.4	0.4*
75 - 84	1.5	2.0	1.0	1.4	2.0	1.0	2.1	2.4*	1.8*
85 & over	1.4	2.2	0.9*	1.4	2.3	0.8*	1.9*	1.1*	2.5*

Table 38

Percent distribution of deaths from all nontransport accidents
and specified types of nontransport accidents, by place of occurrence:
United States, 1959-61

Type of accident	Total[a]	Home (.0)	Farm (.1)	Mine and quarry (.2)	Industrial place and premises (.3)	Place for recreation and sport (.4)	Street and highway (.5)	Public building (.6)	Resident insti- tution (.7)	Other specified places (.8)
Total nontransport accidents (E870-E936)	100.0	56.2	5.8	1.4	5.7	1.6	4.4	3.2	8.0	13.6
Falls (E900-E904)	100.0	64.6	1.3	0.2	3.0	0.5	6.3	4.3	16.0	3.9
Fire and explosion (E916)	100.0	85.2	1.8	0.4	4.4	0.2	0.7	2.8	2.0	2.4
Drowning (E929)	100.0	9.8	7.6	2.2	1.0	8.5	0.1	0.5	0.4	70.0
Firearm (E919)	100.0	55.7	13.7	0.9	1.1	0.9	5.7	3.5	0.1	18.3
Machinery (E912)	100.0	4.3	47.2	4.0	27.9	0.9	6.4	1.7	0.3	7.2
Poisoning by solid and liquid sub- stances (E870-E888)	100.0	85.2	1.7	-	1.5	0.2	1.4	3.7	3.0	3.3
Poisoning by gases and vapors (E890-E895)	100.0	69.6	2.2	0.5	6.7	0.8	7.1	5.7	0.3	7.0

[a] Excludes place not specified.

Table 39
Death rates for homicide, by age, color, and sex:
United States, 1959-61
(E964, E980-E984)

Age	Total			White			Nonwhite		
	Total	Male	Female	Total	Male	Female	Total	Male	Female
All ages	4.7	7.0	2.4	2.5	3.6	1.5	21.3	34.0	9.4
Under 1	4.4	4.6	4.2	3.5	3.7	3.3	9.7	9.9	9.4
1	1.2	1.3	1.2	0.9	0.9	0.9	3.0	3.2	2.8
2	1.0	0.9	1.0	0.8	0.8	0.8	2.1	1.9*	2.3
3	0.7	0.7	0.7	0.7	0.6	0.7	1.1*	1.0*	1.2*
4	0.5	0.7	0.4	0.5	0.7	0.3*	0.8*	0.7*	0.8*
5 - 14	0.5	0.6	0.5	0.4	0.5	0.4	1.1	1.4	0.9
15 - 24	5.8	8.9	2.7	2.8	4.2	1.5	27.1	43.9	11.5
25 - 34	9.4	14.3	4.7	4.1	5.9	2.3	49.5	81.4	21.9
35 - 44	8.1	12.2	4.1	3.9	5.5	2.3	44.0	71.6	19.2
45 - 54	6.1	9.6	2.8	3.5	5.2	1.9	30.0	50.7	10.3
55 - 64	4.1	6.6	1.7	2.7	4.2	1.3	17.7	29.7	6.1
65 - 74	2.9	4.7	1.3	2.2	3.4	1.1	10.9	19.4	3.2
75 - 84	2.6	3.9	1.6	2.1	2.9	1.5	9.3	16.0	3.4*
85 & over	2.6	3.8	1.8	2.0	2.5	1.6	9.8	17.0*	4.1*
Age-adjusted									
Total	5.2	7.8	2.6	2.7	3.9	1.5	25.2	41.3	10.7
Under 15	0.8	0.9	0.8	0.6	0.8	0.6	1.8	2.0	1.6
65 & over	2.8	4.5	1.4	2.2	3.2	1.2	10.5	18.4	3.3

Table 40

Death rates for homicide, by age, color, and sex,
for metropolitan and nonmetropolitan counties: United States, 1959-61
(E964, E980-E984)

| | White | | | | | Nonwhite | | | | |
| | | Metropolitan counties | | | Non-metro-politan counties | | | Metropolitan counties | | Non-metro-politan counties |
Age and sex	Total	Total	with central city	without central city		Total	Total	with central city	without central city	
Males	3.6	3.5	3.9	2.1	3.7	34.0	35.7	36.7	25.5	30.9
Under 1	3.7	4.3	4.6	3.1	2.6	9.9	13.3	14.0	6.2*	3.9*
1-4	0.8	0.9	0.9	0.6*	0.6	1.7	1.9	2.1	-	1.4*
5-14	0.5	0.5	0.5	0.5	0.4	1.4	1.6	1.7	1.1*	1.1
15-24	4.2	4.5	5.1	2.3	3.6	43.9	46.7	48.4	30.3	39.8
25-34	5.9	5.6	6.2	3.2	6.6	81.4	78.5	80.5	57.7	88.6
35-44	5.5	5.1	5.9	2.7	6.3	71.6	69.7	71.6	49.1	76.2
45-54	5.2	4.6	4.9	3.2	6.3	50.7	50.3	51.0	42.5	51.3
55-64	4.2	4.0	4.2	3.1	4.7	29.7	29.9	30.8	20.3	29.4
65-74	3.4	3.4	3.6	2.2	3.4	19.4	20.3	20.0	23.2*	18.3
75-84	2.9	3.1	3.2	2.7*	2.6	16.0	16.1	16.9	8.9*	15.9
85 & over	2.5	2.9*	3.3*	1.1*	2.1*	17.0*	24.1*	26.9*	-	10.3*
Age-adjusted										
Total	3.9	3.7	4.1	2.3	4.1	41.3	41.2	42.3	29.9	42.1
Under 15	0.8	0.8	0.8	0.7	0.6	2.0	2.4	2.6	1.1*	1.3
65 & over	3.2	3.3	3.5	2.3	3.1	18.4	19.4	19.5	18.6	17.4
Females	1.5	1.5	1.6	1.0	1.4	9.4	9.9	10.1	7.1	8.5
Under 1	3.3	3.8	4.1	2.7*	2.4	9.4	11.9	12.2	8.1*	5.1*
1-4	0.7	0.8	0.8	0.7	0.5	1.8	2.2	2.4	-	1.0*
5-14	0.4	0.4	0.4	0.3*	0.4	0.9	1.0	1.1	0.5*	0.6*
15-24	0.7	1.5	1.6	1.1	1.5	11.5	11.6	12.0	7.5*	11.2
25-34	1.5	2.2	2.4	1.4	2.4	21.9	21.0	21.6	14.2	24.0
35-44	2.3	2.2	2.5	1.3	2.4	19.2	19.0	19.2	17.2	19.7
45-54	1.9	1.9	2.0	1.1	2.1	10.3	10.0	10.2	7.5*	10.9
55-64	1.3	1.3	1.4	0.8	1.2	6.1	6.4	6.5	5.2*	5.7
65-74	1.1	1.2	1.2	1.3	1.0	3.2	2.8	2.9	1.5*	3.7
75-84	1.5	1.7	1.8	1.1*	1.3	3.4*	3.6*	3.5*	3.9*	3.1*
85 & over	1.6	1.7*	1.8*	1.2*	1.6*	4.1*	6.2*	3.4*	33.5*	1.8*
Age-adjusted										
Total	1.5	1.5	1.7	1.0	1.6	10.7	10.6	10.8	7.8	10.9
Under 15	0.6	0.7	0.7	0.5	0.5	1.6	2.0	2.2	0.8*	1.0
65 & over	1.2	1.3	1.4	1.2	1.1	3.3	3.1	3.1	3.4*	3.5

Table 41   Age-adjusted death rates for homicide, persons age 15 and over,
by color, sex, and marital status: United States, 1959-61
(E964, E980-E984)

Age and marital status	Total			White			Nonwhite		
	Total	Male	Female	Total	Male	Female	Total	Male	Female
15 & over									
Total	6.6	10.2	3.2	3.3	4.9	1.8	33.2	55.0	13.6
Single	10.7	16.3	3.2	4.5	7.1	1.1	50.2	74.3	15.3
Married	5.4	8.6	3.0	2.8	4.2	1.8	28.0	47.9	13.1
Widowed	19.9	48.2	13.2	8.2	14.8	6.5	51.1	139.9	30.6
Divorced	21.5	39.2	10.6	15.9	27.9	8.3	57.9	122.2	23.5
15 - 64									
Total	7.0	10.8	3.4	3.5	5.1	1.9	35.5	58.6	14.7
Single	11.4	17.2	3.4	4.6	7.3	1.1	53.8	79.2	16.9
Married	5.7	9.2	3.2	2.9	4.4	1.8	29.8	51.4	14.1
Widowed	21.6	52.3	14.4	8.8	15.8	7.1	55.4	151.5	33.4
Divorced	22.9	41.7	11.4	16.8	29.6	8.9	60.8	129.2	25.4
65 & over									
Total	2.8	4.6	1.4	2.2	3.3	1.2	10.5	18.7	3.3
Single	3.7	6.9	1.1	3.1	5.5	1.1	14.5	25.3	0.0*
Married	2.4	3.0	1.4	1.8	2.2	1.3	9.3	13.2	2.2*
Widowed	2.8	7.7	1.4	2.1	5.4	1.2	9.0	24.4	3.7
Divorced	8.4	14.6	2.6*	6.5	11.1	2.4*	29.0	52.3	4.1*

Table 42   Age-adjusted death rates for homicide, white persons,
by sex and nativity: United States and each geographic division, 1959-61
(E964, E980-E984)

Geographic area	Both sexes			Male			Female		
	Total	Native	Foreign	Total	Native	Foreign	Total	Native	Foreign
United States	2.7	2.6	2.6	3.8	3.7	4.0	1.5	1.5	1.4
New England	1.2	1.2	0.8	1.4	1.4	0.4*	1.0	0.9	1.0*
Middle Atlantic	1.7	1.4	2.1	2.4	1.8	2.8	1.1	0.9	1.4
East North Central	2.0	1.9	3.0	2.8	2.6	4.8	1.3	1.2	1.3
West North Central	1.8	1.8	2.1	2.4	2.4	3.1	1.2	1.2	1.0*
South Atlantic	3.8	3.7	2.2	5.6	5.5	2.2	2.1	2.1	2.0*
East South Central	4.7	4.6	2.8*	7.7	7.7	5.0*	1.8	1.7	0.9*
West South Central	4.4	4.2	7.5	6.9	6.6	13.3	2.0	2.0	2.7*
Mountain	3.8	3.7	4.2	5.2	5.0	5.7	2.4	2.4	2.7*
Pacific	3.0	2.9	2.9	4.1	3.9	4.7	1.9	1.9	1.3

Table 43   Age-adjusted death rates for homicide, by color and sex:
United States, each geographic division and state, 1959-61
(E964, E980-E984)

Geographic area	Total			White			Nonwhite		
	Total	Male	Female	Total	Male	Female	Total	Male	Female
United States	5.2	7.8	2.6	2.7	3.9	1.5	25.2	41.3	10.7
New England	1.5	1.7	1.2	1.2	1.4	1.0	9.9	11.5	8.2
Connecticut	1.7	2.0	1.4	1.1	1.4	0.9	13.4	14.7	12.3
Maine	1.8	2.0	1.6	1.8	2.0	1.7	-	-	-
Massachusetts	1.3	1.6	1.0	1.1	1.3	0.9	7.8	10.4*	5.3*
New Hampshire	1.2	1.5*	0.9*	1.2	1.5*	0.9*	-	-	-
Rhode Island	1.4	1.6	1.1*	1.3	1.5*	1.0*	7.8*	\7.9*	7.7*
Vermont	0.9*	1.3*	0.7*	0.9*	1.3*	0.7*	-	-	-
Middle Atlantic	3.2	4.8	1.7	1.7	2.4	1.1	18.8	31.3	8.1
New Jersey	2.7	3.7	1.7	1.4	1.8	1.0	15.6	23.7	8.2
New York	3.7	5.9	1.7	2.0	3.0	1.0	19.6	33.9	7.5
Pennsylvania	2.8	3.9	1.8	1.4	1.7	1.1	19.3	31.1	8.9
East North Central	3.9	5.9	2.1	2.0	2.8	1.3	25.1	40.7	10.7
Illinois	5.2	8.2	2.3	2.5	3.7	1.3	28.2	47.7	10.7
Indiana	3.5	5.5	1.6	2.0	2.9	1.1	27.8	48.2	9.3
Michigan	3.9	5.6	2.2	2.0	2.7	1.3	21.8	33.7	10.5
Ohio	3.7	5.3	2.3	1.9	2.5	1.4	24.1	37.7	11.7
Wisconsin	1.7	2.0	1.4	1.4	1.5	1.2	15.6	21.3	9.8*
West North Central	2.9	4.2	1.6	1.8	2.4	1.2	29.0	48.5	11.4
Iowa	1.3	1.4	1.1	1.1	1.3	1.0	10.4*	17.5*	3.8*
Kansas	2.8	3.6	2.0	1.9	2.2	1.7	20.3	32.2	8.1*
Minnesota	1.4	2.1	0.8	1.2	1.8	0.6	17.7*	23.4*	11.4*
Missouri	5.7	8.8	2.7	3.0	4.3	1.7	32.8	57.1	12.0
Nebraska	2.5	3.7	1.4	1.4	1.8	1.1	42.2	74.3	10.4*
North Dakota	1.4	1.9*	0.8*	0.8	1.2*	0.4*	30.4*	40.6*	21.1*
South Dakota	2.2	2.5	1.9*	1.4	1.5*	1.2*	25.4*	35.3*	15.4*
South Atlantic	9.2	14.1	4.5	3.8	5.5	2.1	29.3	47.3	13.0
Delaware	4.9	6.6	3.3	2.2	2.7*	1.6*	23.2	32.5	13.9*
District of Columbia	11.2	16.9	6.1	4.1	6.2	2.4*	17.0	26.2	8.8
Florida	10.9	16.2	5.8	3.9	5.3	2.6	43.4	67.8	20.2
Georgia	12.1	19.1	5.6	4.6	7.0	2.4	33.9	57.1	14.2
Maryland	5.6	8.0	3.2	2.4	3.2	1.7	21.6	33.3	10.5
North Carolina	10.2	16.5	4.2	4.1	6.6	1.7	31.5	52.4	12.8
South Carolina	10.6	16.5	4.9	4.4	6.6	2.3	24.9	41.4	10.6
Virginia	7.5	11.0	4.0	3.8	5.2	2.4	23.0	36.1	10.6
West Virginia	4.4	6.8	2.1	3.7	5.9	1.6	19.7	29.0	12.1*
East South Central	9.6	15.8	3.7	4.7	7.7	1.8	29.3	50.9	11.2
Alabama	11.8	19.5	4.6	4.8	7.9	1.9	30.9	54.4	11.5
Kentucky	7.7	12.7	2.9	5.7	9.7	1.9	34.7	54.6	16.4
Mississippi	11.3	18.6	4.5	3.5	5.3	1.7	24.7	43.5	9.1
Tennessee	8.1	13.3	3.2	4.2	6.9	1.6	30.6	52.9	11.9
West South Central	8.3	13.4	3.4	4.4	6.9	2.0	29.8	51.7	10.6
Arkansas	8.2	13.5	3.3	3.8	6.1	1.6	27.9	49.4	10.4
Louisiana	9.3	14.9	4.1	3.3	4.9	1.9	23.9	41.1	9.3
Oklahoma	5.6	8.9	2.4	3.7	5.7	1.7	26.3	45.6	9.7
Texas	8.6	13.9	3.4	5.0	7.8	2.2	35.4	61.6	11.8
Mountain	4.9	7.0	2.9	3.8	5.2	2.4	27.8	42.7	12.1
Arizona	7.1	10.6	3.5	4.8	7.1	2.4	31.0	47.2	14.0
Colorado	4.7	6.7	2.8	3.8	5.2	2.4	33.0	51.3	14.1*
Idaho	2.3	2.5	2.1*	2.0	1.9*	2.0*	26.2*	40.8*	8.5*
Montana	3.9	5.4	2.4	3.3	4.4	2.3	21.6*	34.2*	8.0*
Nevada	8.6	11.5	5.4	6.4	7.8	4.7*	40.5	62.0*	16.8*
New Mexico	6.6	9.4	3.8	5.8	8.3	3.3	17.4	24.9	9.1*
Utah	1.9	2.5	1.3*	1.7	2.2	1.3*	9.7*	18.3*	-
Wyoming	4.4	6.3	2.5*	3.4	4.5	2.3*	51.6*	90.6*	11.0*
Pacific	4.1	5.7	2.5	3.0	4.1	1.9	14.7	21.5	7.6
Alaska	9.2	11.1	6.7*	7.2	9.6	3.8*	19.1	19.6*	18.5*
California	4.4	6.2	2.7	3.3	4.4	2.1	17.7	26.2	8.9
Hawaii	3.0	3.9	1.9*	1.9*	2.6*	0.9*	3.5	4.4	2.3*
Oregon	2.6	3.8	1.5	2.0	2.7	1.3	30.8	52.2	8.1*
Washington	2.7	3.9	1.6	2.2	3.0	1.3	18.0	25.4	8.4*

Table 44

Percent distribution of deaths from homicide,
by month of occurrence, and age: United States, 1959-61
(E964, E980-E984)

Month	All ages	Under 5	5-14	15-24	25-34	35-44	45-54	55-64	65-74	75-84	85 & over
Total	100.0	100.0	100.0	100.0	100.0	100.0	100.0	100.0	100.0	100.0	100.0*
January	8.1	9.5	9.5	8.0	8.3	8.0	8.3	6.7	7.5	9.1	4.2
February	7.1	7.5	7.3	6.5	7.6	6.9	7.0	7.3	6.9	8.0	12.5
March	7.8	7.4	8.1	7.5	7.4	8.0	7.6	8.5	8.5	10.5	5.6
April	7.7	9.2	7.0	7.3	7.2	8.3	7.6	8.5	6.6	6.6	12.5
May	8.2	7.5	7.3	7.8	8.6	7.9	8.1	8.8	9.4	7.5	6.9
June	8.0	7.7	7.0	8.2	7.9	8.4	7.8	7.4	8.4	6.1	5.6
July	9.2	7.6	7.9	10.3	9.6	9.3	8.6	8.5	9.3	6.9	11.1
August	9.5	9.3	12.4	9.7	9.3	9.4	9.8	8.6	9.6	8.0	5.6
September	8.5	7.8	10.0	8.8	8.6	8.2	8.2	9.1	8.9	8.3	6.9
October	8.4	9.2	6.5	8.1	8.7	8.1	8.4	9.3	7.1	8.3	9.7
November	8.5	8.6	9.1	8.6	8.1	8.5	9.4	7.6	9.1	8.6	6.9
December	9.1	8.8	7.9	9.4	8.7	9.0	9.3	9.8	8.6	11.9	12.5

Table 45   Number of persons injured per 1,000 population, by demographic
           characteristics and severity of injury: United States,
           July 1959-June 1961

Characteristics	Total persons injured	Persons with:			
		Medically attended injuries	Activity-restricting injuries	Bed-disabling injuries	Hospitalized injuries
All persons	255.2	213.7	150.1	58.0	11.2
Sex					
Male	301.2	260.9	169.3	64.8	14.5
Female	211.7	168.9	131.9	51.6	8.1
Age					
0-14	303.8	254.8	169.4	66.4	11.0
15-24	291.6	259.5	171.1	55.0	9.5
25-44	227.8	190.8	134.7	52.8	11.2
45-64	218.3	183.8	133.3	55.0	11.4
65 & over	189.5	131.1	132.5	54.3	14.2
Color					
White	260.9	219.5	151.0	56.6	10.3
Nonwhite	211.4	168.4	143.1	68.6	18.3
Family income					
Under $2,000	229.5	165.8	157.3	60.6	11.1
$2,000-3,999	253.3	213.3	160.7	61.2	8.5
$4,000-6,999	263.9	224.8	149.9	59.7	12.6
$7,000 & over	258.2	222.0	140.3	52.5	12.2
Unknown	256.7	223.6	142.1	54.9	*
Region					
Northeast	232.5	205.7	122.3	49.1	11.4
North Central	260.2	218.1	150.1	52.3	11.4
South	243.2	195.7	154.1	63.0	8.7
West	308.5	254.6	189.7	74.3	15.6
Usual activity status					
Preschool and school	306.6	259.1	173.1	66.7	11.2
Working	253.6	221.4	145.7	58.8	14.6
Keeping house	181.7	138.6	118.8	40.6	7.0
Retired	191.5	137.2	147.8	78.3	*
Other	255.9	206.6	151.4	50.5	*

Table 46   Number of persons injured per 1,000 population, by demographic
characteristics and class of accident: United States,
July 1959-June 1961

Characteristics	All classes	Class of accident				
		Moving motor vehicle	Nonmoving motor vehicle	Work	Home	Other
All persons	255.2	16.4	10.7	46.4	106.5	75.3
Sex						
Male	301.2	18.8	13.4	82.2	98.5	88.3
Female	211.7	14.1	8.1	12.4	114.0	63.1
Age						
0-14	303.8	9.3	10.9	...	168.5	115.1
15-24	291.6	30.0	12.2	60.8	61.1	127.5
25-44	227.8	17.2	11.8	81.1	73.7	44.0
45-64	218.3	18.8	7.3	77.8	78.0	36.3
65 & over	189.5	13.7	11.9	18.3	110.9	34.7
Color						
White	260.9	15.9	10.7	46.3	109.7	78.3
Nonwhite	211.4	20.0	10.7	46.5	81.9	52.4
Family income						
Under $2,000	229.5	14.8	10.6	34.3	98.3	71.5
$2,000-3,999	253.3	10.5	11.8	52.1	111.1	67.7
$4,000-6,999	263.9	21.6	9.9	53.0	108.0	71.5
$7,000 & over	258.2	16.4	12.3	38.0	108.6	83.0
Unknown	256.7	*	*	51.4	92.7	98.7
Region						
Northeast	232.5	14.2	6.1	37.3	95.5	79.4
North Central	260.2	16.5	9.6	54.3	100.9	79.0
South	243.2	10.4	12.9	45.6	111.3	63.0
West	308.5	31.7	16.2	48.5	126.2	86.0
Usual activity status						
Preschool and school	306.6	10.5	10.6	...	160.1	125.5
Working	253.6	21.4	14.2	121.3	56.8	39.9
Keeping house	181.7	16.2	5.9	5.9	106.4	47.3
Retired	191.5	*	*	19.4	122.2	37.4
Other	255.9	29.5	*	35.9	71.3	110.0

Table 47   Number of bed-disability days per 1,000 population, by
demographic characteristics and class of accident:
United States, July 1959-June 1961

| Characteristics | Class of accident | | | | | |
	All classes	Moving motor vehicle	Nonmoving motor vehicle	Work	Home	Other
All persons	644.0	145.9	19.7	137.2	211.4	129.8
Sex						
Male	686.1	165.4	25.3	216.4	128.4	150.5
Female	604.2	127.4	14.3	62.1	290.0	110.3
Age						
0-14	272.4	38.4	2.8	...	126.9	104.3
15-24	387.0	128.3	*	45.9	79.5	133.4
25-44	683.9	176.8	34.1	210.4	147.2	115.4
45-64	988.8	247.4	36.7	325.7	253.4	125.6
65 & over	1471.0	238.0	28.8	128.3	813.0	271.0
Color						
White	615.4	146.1	19.4	123.2	208.7	118.0
Nonwhite	865.7	144.1	22.0	245.6	232.3	221.7
Family income						
Under $2,000	1150.1	245.2	21.7	200.9	412.8	269.4
$2,000-3,999	740.7	194.3	48.0	190.8	188.4	119.2
$4,000-6,999	558.4	128.6	10.8	116.1	187.3	115.5
$7,000 & over	389.5	90.8	8.8	84.0	130.5	75.4
Unknown	746.9	94.9	19.4	162.6	309.9	160.2
Region						
Northeast	461.3	108.0	17.7	84.6	145.1	105.9
North Central	536.6	143.5	21.9	82.4	145.5	143.3
South	778.1	147.1	20.4	182.6	289.5	138.6
West	892.4	212.8	17.4	240.2	294.2	127.9
Usual activity status						
Preschool and school	295.7	42.0	2.6	...	134.7	116.4
Working	664.2	177.6	36.0	271.8	86.4	92.4
Keeping house	624.9	142.1	8.6	45.9	300.0	128.4
Retired	2183.8	373.9	45.7	239.5	1102.3	422.5
Other	1809.5	471.3	50.1	431.6	586.4	270.2

Table 48   Average annual number of persons injured, number with
            activity-restricting injuries, and number per 1,000
            population, by age, sex, and color: United States,
            July 1959-June 1961

Age and sex	Number of persons injured (in thousands)			Persons injured per 1,000 population		
	Total	White	Nonwhite	Total	White	Nonwhite
Persons injured						
Total	44,995	40,731	4,264	255.2	260.9	211.4
Age						
0-14	17,127	15,703	1,424	303.8	324.0	179.8
15-24	6,759	6,117	642	291.6	302.2	218.6
25-44	10,346	9,220	1,126	227.8	227.5	229.9
45-64	7,856	7,072	783	218.3	216.6	234.2
65 & over	2,906	2,618	288	189.5	183.6	268.7
Sex						
Male	25,835	23,182	2,653	301.2	304.8	273.1
Female	19,160	17,549	1,611	211.7	219.2	154.1
Persons injured with restricted activity						
Total	26,465	23,578	2,887	150.1	151.0	143.1
Age						
0-14	9,552	8,567	985	169.4	176.8	124.4
15-24	3,966	3,546	420	171.1	175.2	143.0
25-44	6,120	5,396	724	134.7	133.1	147.8
45-64	4,796	4,237	559	133.3	129.8	167.2
65 & over	2,031	1,831	199	132.5	128.4	185.6
Sex						
Male	14,524	12,776	1,748	169.3	168.0	179.9
Female	11,941	10,802	1,139	131.9	134.9	108.9

Table 49   Number of persons injured and number with activity-
restricting injuries per 1,000 population, by age, sex, and
marital status: United States, July 1959-June 1961

	Persons injured per 1,000 population				
	Total		17 and over		
Age and sex	marital	Under		Never	
	status	17	Married	married	Other
Persons injured					
Total	255.2	306.6	222.3	251.7	227.2
Age					
0-16	306.6	306.6	...	...	...
17-24	277.9	...	250.0	298.3	247.3
25-44	227.8	...	229.8	214.5	217.3
45-64	218.3	...	221.0	154.3	231.6
65 & over	189.5	...	166.4	142.9	226.5
Sex					
Male	301.2	350.8	265.4	311.6	248.1
Female	211.7	260.7	179.8	178.6	220.0
Persons injured					
with restricted					
activity					
Total	150.1	173.1	133.7	141.3	155.5
Age					
0-16	173.1	173.1	...	...	...
17-24	158.7	...	140.7	174.1	90.3
25-44	134.7	...	135.5	109.0	159.5
45-64	133.3	...	133.7	84.5	152.6
65 & over	132.5	...	119.2	61.8	160.8
Sex					
Male	169.3	194.0	150.0	172.8	162.9
Female	131.9	151.4	117.6	102.7	152.9

Table 50   Number of persons injured and number with activity-
            restricting injuries per 1,000 population, by age, sex, and
            family income: United States, July 1959-June 1961

Age and sex	Persons injured per 1,000 population					
	All incomes	Under $1,999	$2,000-3,999	$4,000-6,999	$7,000 & over	Unknown
Persons injured						
Total	255.2	229.5	253.3	263.9	258.2	256.7
Age						
0-14	303.8	233.0	277.7	308.6	339.5	347.2
15-24	291.6	314.8	319.7	269.0	281.7	293.0
25-44	227.8	225.7	253.9	223.8	205.8	298.9
45-64	218.3	187.4	198.7	251.7	217.3	195.2
65 & over	189.5	213.3	191.3	196.5	177.1	90.0
Sex						
Male	301.2	251.1	311.0	313.7	295.0	327.8
Female	211.7	211.7	200.6	214.5	221.4	192.6
Persons injured with restricted activity						
Total	150.1	157.3	160.7	149.9	140.3	142.1
Age						
0-14	169.4	188.1	161.8	159.3	183.3	172.1
15-24	171.1	160.0	202.9	169.4	142.9	204.1
25-44	134.7	162.1	163.2	132.1	111.6	148.4
45-64	133.3	133.3	137.5	150.5	115.2	119.5
65 & over	132.5	141.4	138.8	135.0	149.9	50.4
Sex						
Male	169.3	157.8	198.2	166.9	156.0	173.2
Female	131.9	156.9	126.5	133.0	124.5	114.1

Table 51   Number of persons injured and number with activity-restricting injuries per 1,000 population, by age, sex, and usual activity: United States, July 1959-June 1961

Age and sex	Persons injured per 1,000 population					
	All activities	Preschool and school[a]	Working	Keeping house	Retired[a]	Other[a]
Persons injured						
Total	255.2	306.6	253.6	181.7	191.5	255.9
Age						
0-16	306.6	306.6	...	...	...	...
17-24	277.9	...	317.1	166.7	...	292.2
25-44	227.8	...	249.3	186.8	...	245.9
45-64	218.3	...	235.4	196.8	217.2	107.9
65 & over	189.5	...	268.4	151.3	188.0	227.4
Sex						
Male	301.2	350.8	283.3	...	150.7	296.0
Female	211.7	260.7	185.9	181.7	383.6	185.8
Persons injured with restricted activity						
Total	150.1	173.1	145.7	118.8	147.8	151.4
Age						
0-16	173.1	173.1	...	...	...	...
17-24	158.7	...	184.4	75.8	...	173.6
25-44	134.7	...	139.1	126.2	...	140.0
45-64	133.3	...	136.3	132.4	190.7	55.1
65 & over	132.5	...	181.2	100.2	141.9	153.7
Sex						
Male	169.3	194.0	157.0	...	123.1	166.5
Female	131.9	151.4	119.9	118.8	264.0	125.0

[a]Preschool and school - under 17 years; retired - 45 years and over; other - 17 years and over.

Table 52   Number of persons injured and number with activity-restricting
            injuries per 1,000 population, by age, sex, and education of
            family head: United States, July 1959-June 1961

Age and sex	Persons injured per 1,000 population					
	All education groups	0-4 years	5-8 years	9-12 years	College	Unknown
Persons injured						
Total	255.2	201.3	233.6	275.5	271.8	168.5
Age						
0-16	306.6	175.1	243.5	334.7	366.0	237.1
17-24	277.9	183.5	279.7	301.7	269.5	56.0
25-44	227.8	357.2	217.6	235.9	203.1	113.3
45-64	218.3	189.4	222.0	218.7	228.9	197.0
65 & over	189.5	134.8	227.9	185.9	165.0	117.3
Sex						
Male	301.2	264.1	287.5	315.3	317.9	194.5
Female	211.7	140.3	182.0	238.3	227.6	143.8
Persons injured with restricted activity						
Total	150.1	160.6	148.1	154.9	146.4	89.7
Age						
0-16	173.1	151.3	156.6	182.8	184.9	102.7
17-24	158.7	183.5	191.2	155.0	135.7	*
25-44	134.7	281.7	135.6	132.4	112.6	94.8
45-64	133.3	119.7	133.1	135.6	140.5	110.0
65 & over	132.5	113.1	148.8	136.8	115.3	73.3
Sex						
Male	169.3	207.0	175.5	169.5	155.1	98.8
Female	131.9	115.3	121.8	141.2	138.0	81.1

Table 53 Number of persons injured and number with activity-
restricting injuries per 1,000 population by age, sex, and
living arrangements: United States, July 1959-June 1961

Age and sex	Persons injured per 1,000 population			
	All arrange-ments	Living alone or with non-relatives	Married, living with relatives	Other, living with relatives
Persons injured				
Total	255.2	275.0	222.9	284.3
Age				
0-16	306.6	734.4	...	305.7
17-24	277.9	430.2	252.0	268.3
25-44	227.8	242.0	230.1	202.1
45-64	218.3	220.5	222.1	188.4
65 & over	189.5	261.9	165.6	167.7
Sex				
Male	301.2	338.0	266.5	331.7
Female	211.7	231.4	179.8	239.2
Persons injured with restricted activity				
Total	150.1	153.2	133.6	165.9
Age				
0-16	173.1	242.2	...	173.0
17-24	158.7	172.0	140.8	169.8
25-44	134.7	130.0	135.2	133.1
45-64	133.3	133.2	134.1	127.1
65 & over	132.5	175.3	118.0	120.5
Sex				
Male	169.3	154.2	150.3	190.2
Female	131.9	152.5	117.2	142.9

Table 54   Average annual number of persons injured and number per
1,000 population, by sex, class of accident, and color:
United States, July 1959-June 1961

Sex and class of accident	Number of persons injured (in thousands)			Persons injured per 1,000 population		
	Total	White	Non-white	Total	White	Non-white
Both sexes						
All classes	44,995	40,731	4,264	255.2	260.9	211.4
Moving motor-vehicle	2,890	2,486	404	16.4	15.9	20.0
Nonmoving motor-vehicle	1,881	1,665	216	10.7	10.7	10.7
Work	8,172	7,235	937	46.4	46.3	46.5
Home	18,772	17,121	1,651	106.5	109.7	81.9
Other	13,281	12,224	1,057	75.3	78.3	52.4
Male						
All classes	25,835	23,182	2,653	301.2	304.8	273.1
Moving motor-vehicle	1,613	1,318	295	18.8	17.3	30.4
Nonmoving motor-vehicle	1,147	950	197	13.4	12.5	20.3
Work	7,054	6,256	797	82.2	82.2	82.0
Home	8,448	7,733	715	98.5	101.7	73.6
Other	7,572	6,924	648	88.3	91.0	66.7
Female						
All classes	19,160	17,549	1,611	211.7	219.2	154.1
Moving motor-vehicle	1,276	1,168	109	14.1	14.6	10.4
Nonmoving motor-vehicle	733	715	19	8.1	8.9	1.8
Work	1,118	979	139	12.4	12.2	13.3
Home	10,323	9,388	935	114.0	117.2	89.4
Other	5,708	5,300	409	63.1	66.2	39.1

Table 55   Number of persons injured per 1,000 population, by sex,
           class of accident, and marital status: United States,
           July 1959-June 1961

| Sex and class of accident | Persons injured per 1,000 population | | | | |
| | | | 17 and over | | |
	Total	Under 17	Married	Never married	Other
Both sexes					
All classes	255.2	306.6	222.3	251.7	227.2
Moving motor-vehicle	16.4	10.5	18.4	29.4	14.6
Nonmoving motor-vehicle	10.7	10.6	11.2	8.5	10.7
Work	46.4	...	76.9	67.5	45.4
Home	106.5	160.1	75.2	54.8	116.9
Other	75.3	125.5	40.6	91.6	39.4
Male					
All classes	301.2	350.8	265.4	311.6	248.1
Moving motor-vehicle	18.8	12.2	18.9	37.7	24.8
Nonmoving motor-vehicle	13.4	12.0	15.4	11.2	8.0
Work	82.2	...	138.2	100.4	117.5
Home	98.5	173.9	55.9	44.0	68.1
Other	88.3	152.7	37.0	118.1	29.9
Female					
All classes	211.7	260.7	179.8	178.6	220.0
Moving motor-vehicle	14.1	8.6	17.9	19.3	11.1
Nonmoving motor-vehicle	8.1	9.1	7.0	5.1	11.7
Work	12.4	...	16.4	27.1	20.8
Home	114.0	145.7	94.3	68.0	133.6
Other	63.1	97.2	44.1	59.1	42.7

Table 56 Number of persons injured per 1,000 population, by sex, class of accident, and education of family head: United States, July 1959-June 1961

Sex and class of accident	Persons injured per 1,000 population					
	Total	0-4 years	5-8 years	9-12 years	College	Unknown
Both sexes						
All classes	255.2	201.3	233.6	275.5	271.8	168.5
Moving motor-vehicle	16.4	10.2	15.3	16.3	20.4	18.6
Nonmoving motor-vehicle	10.7	7.0	9.3	12.6	10.4	3.6
Work	46.4	58.1	55.9	49.7	20.0	40.1
Home	106.5	81.7	92.9	112.9	129.0	53.3
Other	75.3	44.4	60.3	84.0	92.0	53.1
Male						
All classes	301.2	264.1	287.5	315.3	317.9	194.5
Moving motor-vehicle	18.8	11.8	19.1	16.1	27.9	17.6
Nonmoving motor-vehicle	13.4	11.3	12.2	15.4	12.0	7.3
Work	82.2	106.0	105.9	85.8	30.6	66.1
Home	98.5	88.9	76.1	103.3	135.8	24.0
Other	88.3	46.1	74.3	94.7	111.7	79.0
Female						
All classes	211.7	140.3	182.0	238.3	227.6	143.8
Moving motor-vehicle	14.1	8.6	11.6	16.4	13.3	19.2
Nonmoving motor-vehicle	8.1	2.9	6.6	10.0	8.9	*
Work	12.4	11.3	8.0	16.0	9.8	15.1
Home	114.0	74.6	108.9	121.9	122.4	81.1
Other	63.1	42.7	46.9	74.0	73.2	28.5

Table 57 Number of persons injured in the labor force per 1,000 persons per year, by occupational group and age: United States, July 1961-June 1963

Occupation group	17 & over	17-24	25-44	45-64	65 & over
All occupation groups	266.4	323.7	284.7	226.1	200.9
Professional, technical, and kindred workers	236.5	203.4	235.5	262.1	147.3
Farmers and farm managers	287.0	438.1	324.5	303.4	122.3
Managers, officials, and proprietors, except farm	168.5	67.9	198.9	136.3	241.9
Clerical and kindred workers	214.7	207.5	255.4	172.6	63.4
Sales workers	175.2	258.0	148.0	186.4	72.9
Craftsmen, foremen, and kindred workers	331.1	513.0	362.5	271.8	105.7
Operatives and kindred workers	331.7	488.7	333.7	234.2	428.6
Private and household workers	228.5	177.6	243.5	224.1	285.1
Service workers, except private household	244.1	367.0	222.3	195.4	311.9
Farm laborers and foremen	306.9	255.5	373.5	303.7	209.3
Laborers, except farm and mine	446.4	470.4	501.4	392.2	118.5
Unknown and new workers[a]	138.7	104.8	218.9	173.2	*

[a]A "new worker" is a person who has a job to which he has not yet reported and has never had a previous job or business.

Table 58 Number of persons injured in the labor force per 1,000
persons per year, by occupational group and class of
accident: United States, July 1961-June 1963

Occupation group	Total	Moving motor-vehicle	Nonmoving motor-vehicle	Work	Home	Other
			Class of accident			
All occupation groups	266.4	24.9	16.2	117.1	76.9	58.5
Professional, technical, and kindred workers	236.5	25.9	8.2	51.7	100.2	58.7
Farmers and farm managers	287.0	7.1	31.9	174.7	89.0	57.9
Managers, officials, and proprietors, except farm	168.5	24.4	21.4	48.6	64.9	36.0
Clerical and kindred workers	214.7	20.2	13.4	42.9	75.5	78.7
Sales workers	175.2	25.7	*	25.0	75.9	53.0
Craftsmen, foremen, and kindred workers	331.1	23.8	22.6	197.8	62.9	56.6
Operatives and kindred workers	331.7	33.7	22.6	186.8	73.8	54.9
Private and household workers	228.5	*	6.0	58.2	154.5	67.2
Service workers, except private household	244.1	28.8	8.9	92.2	63.0	63.6
Farm laborers and fore-men	306.9	34.9	*	177.4	79.8	45.5
Laborers, except farm and mine	446.4	29.0	31.8	306.4	69.9	59.2
Unknown and new workers[a]	138.7	*	*	*	66.8	73.3

[a]A "new worker" is a person who has a job to which he has not yet reported
and has never had a previous job or business.

Table 59   Average annual number of persons injured and number per 1,000
population, by age, sex, and geographic region: United States,
July 1959-June 1961

Age and sex	Region				
	All regions	North-east	North Central	South	West
	Average annual number of persons injured				
All persons	44,995	10,623	13,172	12,935	8,265
Age					
0-14	17,127	4,128	5,227	4,627	3,145
15-24	6,759	1,478	2,125	1,795	1,361
25-44	10,346	2,479	2,818	3,175	1,875
45-64	7,856	1,828	2,270	2,360	1,398
65 & over	2,906	710	732	978	486
Sex					
Male	25,835	6,090	7,863	7,614	4,269
Female	19,160	4,533	5,309	5,321	3,996
	Number injured per 1,000 population				
All persons	255.2	232.5	260.2	243.2	308.5
Age					
0-14	303.8	308.1	319.1	261.1	354.2
15-24	291.6	260.8	325.2	237.5	398.3
25-44	227.8	201.9	218.6	240.9	265.2
45-64	218.3	182.1	222.6	224.9	266.0
65 & over	189.5	165.0	158.5	230.4	224.5
Sex					
Male	301.2	276.2	313.5	297.2	327.8
Female	211.7	191.8	207.8	193.0	290.3

INDEX